# Heart Journey:

## Healing through Encounters with Jesus and Psychology

*A study for women ready for wholeness*

Heart Journey:

Healing through Encounters with Jesus and Psychology

Barbara Lowe

2023© by Barbara Lowe

All rights reserved. Published 2023.

## BIBLE SCRIPTURES

Printed in the United States of America

Spirit Media and our logos are trademarks of Spirit Media

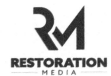

www.restorationmedia.co
9650 Strickland Rd STE 103-111
Raleigh, NC 27615

SPIRIT MEDIA
www.spiritmedia.us
1249 Kildaire Farm Rd STE 112
Cary, NC 27511
1 (888) 800-3744

Kindle Store › Kindle eBooks › Health, Fitness & Dieting
Books › Self-Help › Personal Transformation
Books › Health, Fitness & Dieting › Psychology & Counseling
Books › Christian Books & Bibles › Christian Living

Paperback ISBN: 978-1-961614-15-4
Hardback: 978-1-961614-16-1
Audiobook ISBN: 978-1-961614-17-8
eBook ISBN: 978-1-961614-14-7
Library of Congress Control Number: 2023911416

# Endorsements

In *Heart Journey*™, Dr. Barbara Lowe's expertise in trauma healing shines through as she skillfully guides women on a transformative journey of healing and restoration. This invaluable tool equips individuals to navigate the complexities of their past, offering them a path to deep healing and the restoration of their God-given purpose. This is a groundbreaking resource that weaves together the principles of the Christian faith and the science of trauma healing.

**DR. TIM CLINTON**
*President, American Association of Christian Counselors*

Because virtually everybody, including Christians, has had some kind of trauma in life, there is a great need for sound, Christian resources that explain simply how to get the healing people need. But this book is very special. It is so biblical, so trauma-informed, and so accessible – all in one – written by someone with years of experience working with trauma, it guides readers step-by-step into a comprehensive, yet extremely practical, Christian model of trauma healing.

**ERIC L. JOHNSON, PH.D.**
*Professor of Christian Psychology, Houston Christian University*

Amidst a vast sea of literature, *Heart Journey*™ stands out as a groundbreaking resource that offers a truly unique and transformative approach to personal growth, guiding individuals from soul pain to God-sized purpose. Dr. Lowe's remarkable understanding of the inner world and her ability to lead women on a journey of deep healing and renewal sets her apart in the field.

JON GORDON
*15x Best-Selling Author of The One Truth and The Garden*

*Heart Journey*™ is an exceptional and vital addition to the realms of ministry and psychology. It seamlessly blends a Christian worldview with the science of trauma healing, establishing a solid foundation that is both accessible and practical. I wholeheartedly endorse this book and journal to women within the body of Christ, as it offers profound healing for the heart. Furthermore, I recommend it to my esteemed colleagues as an exemplar of the harmonious integration between our indigenous Christian psychology and the science of trauma healing.

HAROLD G. KOENIG, M.D.
*Professor of Psychiatry and Behavioral Sciences*
*Associate Professor of Medicine*
*Duke University Medical Center, Durham, North Carolina*
*Adjunct Professor, Department of Medicine, King Abdulaziz University, Jeddah, Saudi Arabia*
*Visiting Professor, Shiraz University of Medical Sciences, Shiraz, Iran*
*Editor-in-Chief, International Journal of Psychiatry in Medicine*

Dr. Barbara has given us a powerful gift in *Heart Journey*™. Informed by her experience as a Christian minister and a clinical psychologist, and guided by principles from psychology and neuroscience, *Heart Journey*™ meets each of us at our place of need. Through her conversational tone, Dr. Barbara shares impactful stories, informative teaching, and practical guidance that can transform your life. This book reflects the power of integrating the truths of Scripture, encounters with Jesus, and evidence-based tools that can help each of us heal, grow, and thrive.

NII ADDY, PH.D.
*Yale Neuroscientist, Professor, and Podcast Host*

As a licensed psychologist and Christian minister, Dr. Barbara Lowe understands and affirms both that trauma and unmet psychological needs are widespread in our world and that we are beloved creatures of God, who desires our wholeness and flourishing. While not intended as a substitute for therapy, *Heart Journey*™ is filled to the brim with practical and grounded exercises that can help our hearts unburden from the weight of anxiety and inability to trust in ourselves or others, and to open to a life of freedom and secure rest in God's love. In this hopeful book, Dr. Lowe offers an encouraging pathway to spiritual and psychological restoration and healing.

WARREN KINGHORN, MD, ThD
*Associate Professor of Psychiatry, Duke University Medical Center*
*Esther Colliflower Associate Professor of the Practice of Pastoral and*
*Moral Theology, Duke Divinity School*
*Co-Director, Theology, Medicine, and Culture Initiative, Duke Divinity School*

This book is a timely gift and a rich treasure to the Body of Christ at this time and era of the church and where we find ourselves placed in society today. We have had a huge value in our movement on leaders walking through regular heart healing to unlock the potential God has for them so this heart fruit can filter through a church community. The purpose is that the love of God will be manifested in all that we do in our churches, including how we love and engage our communities, and bring the light of Christ to our cities.

Most of us arrive in adulthood with childhood scars, emotional wounds, and traumas that limit us not only in our relationships with others, but with God our Father Himself. Our own testimony of heart healing and transformation over more than two decades as church Pastors is proof of this, as we have engaged in different forms and models of heart healing and deliverance on a continuous basis.

We have seen the great need for not only psychological theories of transformation but Holy Spirit-inspired, Scripture-filled material that will be tools in the hands of thousands of church leaders, lay leaders, church members, and families placed across every sphere of culture.

We believe that as you deep dive into this book and journal workbook, taking the hand of the Holy Spirit Himself, He wants to walk with you as you unlock the deep places of your heart so that you can become the person you are called to be living your best life in Him!

KATE AND DUNCAN SMITH
*Senior Leaders of Catch the Fire Raleigh*
*Presidents of Catch the Fire World, a global movement of churches,*
*ministry and missions*

Dr. Barbara's skills and giftedness in bringing together psychology, theology, and neuroscience are rare, if not unparalleled. Fortunately, we have a gift and a tool in *Heart Journey*™. Trauma and pain seem ubiquitous, but *Heart Journey*™ is an effective antidote.

Dr. Barbara personally and clinically knows that inner healing is not beyond reach. The all-wise God, who desires wholeness, often uses people who have been "through the valley of tears, only to make it a place of springs" (Psalm 84:6). I highly endorse my friend, Dr. Barbara Lowe, and encourage you to journey forward with her.

RON LEWIS
*Bishop, King's Park churches*
*Every Nation NYC*
*Jordan Lewis Missions*
*Author, Miracles in Manhattan*

In a world where women are yearning for healing, purpose, and restoration, Dr. Barbara Lowe's *Heart Journey*™ book and journal shines as an unyielding beacon of hope. As a woman deeply immersed in both business and ministry, I have had the privilege of witnessing firsthand the remarkable and transformative impact of Dr. Lowe's ministry as a speaker. Time and again, I have seen the profound effectiveness of the *Heart Journey*™ process in the lives of those around me. This extraordinary resource impeccably blends a Christian worldview with the science of trauma healing, providing women with a practical roadmap to embark on a deeply personal and fulfilling journey of inner healing. Without a doubt, this is a must-do study for anyone seeking true transformation.

Within the pages of the *Heart Journey*™ book and journal, Dr. Lowe masterfully integrates psychology with profound encounters with Jesus and the living Word of God. This groundbreaking approach fearlessly calls women to courageously confront their past, release the burdens that weigh them down, and embrace a future overflowing with purpose and meaning. Through the exploration of stability skills, resilience-building practices, narrative examination, and profound heart healing, readers are guided toward experiencing the life-altering power of forgiveness, surrender, and restoration. Dr. Lowe's teachings and insights, deeply rooted in her own life of authenticity and unwavering faith, bear witness to the profound impact of this resource.

If you are a woman yearning to heal the depths of your heart, unlock your true potential, and step into a life of profound significance, the *Heart Journey*™ book and journal are the perfect companions for your sacred journey. Discover the immense power that comes from integrating your faith with psychological healing, and embrace a future that is marked by profound wholeness, unshakable purpose, and a deeper connection with our beloved Savior. Prepare to be transformed as you embark on this extraordinary path toward true healing, restoration, and a life that shines with the radiance of God's love.

LYNETTE LEWIS
*TEDx Speaker*
*Author*
*Business Consultant*
*Pastor's Wife*

Dr. Barbara has written with such great insight! You will be encouraged and inspired to begin your journey toward healing and wholeness. It is a compelling and spirit-filled study book that will make the broken heart thirsty for the healing you long for. It will guide you and quench your thirst with the knowledge imparted to you. Your innermost being will respond with courage as you encounter truth. The inner healing begins as you learn to pour out the pain of your past and find the freedom to live a future that is full, complete, and free indeed in Christ. The truth shared in this book has the power to break the yoke of bondage and set the captive free!

ANNE BEILER
*Founder of Auntie Anne's Pretzels*
*Author and Speaker*

In *Heart Journey*™, Dr. Barbara Lowe guides women on a much-needed journey in trauma healing and the wholeness available in Christ. The heartwork instructions are simple to follow with a lasting and profound impact. This book is a valuable tool for both individuals and clinicians, sharing relevant scientific processes alongside scriptural truths to offer a transformational journey to restore mind-body-spirit well-being.

DR. SAUNDRA DALTON-SMITH
*Bestselling Author of Sacred Rest and Host of I Choose My Best Life*

I am honored to wholeheartedly endorse Dr. Barbara Lowe's integrated *Heart Journey*™ book and journal. As the creator and co-leader of the SOZO inner healing method, I have great anticipation of the powerful impact this book and study guide will have on women of all ages. I am confident that this resource will continue to bring transformative breakthroughs to all who are willing to allow God to remodel and beautify their heart home. I have watched Dr. Barbara gather, empower, and bring whole heart healing to hundreds of women over the past five years I have known her. This book is not only written from a therapist who knows how to fix you but dually from a researched, educated, devoted believer who has allowed God to entirely remodel her own heart home. Roll up your sleeves, get your work clothes on, put your hands to the plow, and be amazed at how God will restore beauty from your life's ashes.

DAWNA DE SILVA
*Bethel Sozo, Co-Leader*
*Author of Sozo: Saved, Healed, Delivered*
*Shifting Atmospheres*
*Atmospheres 101*
*Overcoming Fear*
*Prayers, Declarations, and Strategies*
*Warring with Wisdom*

Often, the challenges we are faced with feel bigger than our blessings and potential. They call into question our peace and our place. Dr. Barbara Lowe's *Heart Journey*™ offers profound insight and practical tools providing the much-needed support that serves to strengthen the foundation our faith is built on. At different times in my life as a young woman of faith, I have longed for such a clear and impactful ministry. It brings me great joy to know that women the world over will now have this life changing place of healing to grow from. I strongly encourage anyone in need of emotional and spiritual wholeness to dive deeply into this phenomenal book. As I tip my hat to this extraordinary woman and this indispensable resource, I am reminded of this bit of Scripture, "Peace I leave you; my peace I give you. I do not give to you as the world gives. Do not let your hearts be troubled and do not be afraid." – John 14:27

LISA KIMMEY WINANS
*Recording Artist*
*Actress*
*Speaker*

*Heart Journey*™ is a beautifully woven synthesis bringing together clinical research with spiritual truths producing a profoundly transformative masterpiece. Dr. Barbara's clinical work and research provide a holistic perspective to honor body, soul, and spirit in a cohesive blend that fosters sustainable healing. The *Heart Journey*™ book and workbook seamlessly walk the reader through a process that fosters past healing and empowers participants to live fullheartedly from their true selves into their life purpose. A true treasure that has exquisite value that will benefit everyone!

DR. SHANNAN CRAWFORD
*Licensed Psychologist*
*Executive Coach*
*Speaker*

When it comes to healing the matters of the heart, it is of utmost importance to seek guidance from one who has answered the call of Jesus—one who knows Jesus, one with heart-healing experience, one whose leadership can be trusted, one who has your best in mind. Dr. Barbara Lowe is that one. She is one I would trust with the matters of my own heart. You can get whole. Dr. Barbara will guide you to healing and wholeness in her deeply insightful and spiritually powerful new book and companion journal—*Heart Journey*™: Healing through Encounters with Jesus & Psychology and *Heart Journey Journal.*

**DR. KIM MAAS**
*Founder/CEO Kim Maas Ministries*
*Author of Prophetic Community: God's Call For All to Minister in His Gifts and The Way of the Kingdom: Seizing the Times For a Great Move of God*

I am honored to offer my enthusiastic endorsement of Dr. Barbara Lowe's groundbreaking book, *Heart Journey*™. As an international speaker, consultant, published author, and Doctor of Theology specializing in Cultural Restoration and Leadership, I have had the privilege of witnessing firsthand the transformative power of Dr. Lowe's teachings. With her exceptional understanding of inner healing and trauma restoration, impeccably blended with a Christian worldview, Dr. Lowe's work in *Heart Journey*™ serves as a beacon of hope for women seeking healing, purpose, and restoration. Her masterful integration of profound encounters with Jesus, the living Word of God, with the principles of inner healing creates a life-altering experience that calls readers to courageously confront and heal from their past, embrace forgiveness, and step into a future overflowing with unshakable faith and profound significance. Prepare to be profoundly transformed as you embark on this extraordinary journey of inner healing guided by Dr. Lowe's expertise and unwavering commitment to empowering women to live lives of wholeness and God-breathed purpose.

**DR. TRACEY STRAWBERRY**
*International Speaker, Consultant, and Trainer*
*Founder of Finding Your Way*
*Author: The Imperfect Marriage, Help for Those Who Think It's Over*
*Author: Clean Sober & Saved Christ-Centered Recovery Curriculums*
*Author Participant: The Invitation to Intimacy with God Devotional*
*Co-Author: Straw, Finding My Way (Biography of Darryl Strawberry)*

In the current age of intense external pressures and unresolved traumas, the levels of confusion and anxiety among adults and children are alarming … even within the Church! In The *Heart Journey*™, Dr. Barbara Lowe has made it possible for you to face the pain that triggers your anxieties. She offers practical tools to effectively apply the Word of God to whatever is driving you. Say goodbye to the empty rhetoric that has shamed you in the past and say hello to your freedom!

BRENDA CROUCH - AUTHOR, SPEAKER, TV HOST

In my sixteen years of pastoring and supporting those with trauma, I haven't found a resource as comprehensive as the *Heart Journey*™ book and the accompanying *Heart Journey*™ *Journal*—the tools, exercises, and biblical truths Dr. Barbara Lowe-Sauve has compiled will bring restoration, wholeness, purpose, and life-long wellness to those who commit to the journey. In addition, participants will have intimate encounters with Jesus and deepen their relationship with Him and others. The *Heart Journey*™ Book and Journal are life-changing resources for individuals and small groups.

VERNA BROWN
*Senior Pastor of Soul Harvest Worship Center*
*Writer*
*Speaker*

*Heart Journey*™ is a comprehensive curriculum which actively addresses and provides practical solutions to the hurt, pain, and disappointments that victims of trauma hide in their hearts. This system is a blueprint of wholeness that was developed on a foundation of biblical principles intertwined with professional psychological insight. God is using Dr. Barbara in supernatural ways to provide healing and restoration to everyone. Her passion exudes from the pages of the book and accompanying journal, giving you practical steps throughout your journey of healing. It addresses your emotional, spiritual and physical recovery needs. I encourage both men and women to be bold enough to take the path of healing and restoration. You owe it to yourself to heal. In doing so, you will experience God's love in ways you never imagined, allowing you to accomplish what you've only dreamed of.

VALORA SHAW-COLE
*Senior Co-Pastor Contagious Church*
*Speaker*
*Author*

*Heart Journey*™ is a game changer for the world. This book is a blueprint with scientific research that helps us better understand the intricacies of the heart and the biblical principles that can help you experience real transformative healing from past trauma. I recommend this book as a resource to guide you through your personal journey to freedom. Every believer should read this book and use it as a tool to help enhance their insight of the inner man and equip them to bring practical healing to the brokenhearted.

ANDY ARGUEZ
*Senior Pastor of Supernatural Culture Church*
*International Speaker*
*Author*
*Senior Ambassador of Philcoin*

Dr. Lowe has created an incredible resource for those trying to heal from a painful past and significant trauma. *The Heart Journey*™ focuses on critical aspects of people's pain that most traditional therapy can ignore altogether or only minimally address. At its foundation, this book and journal allow an intimate relationship with God and spiritual growth in Christ to lead the process of healing and recovery. It is a valuable resource for trauma survivors.

JENNIFER ELLERS, MA
*Institute for Compassionate Care*

I appreciate Dr. Barbara Lowe's ability to integrate Christian psychology, a Biblically-grounded approach to inner healing of the heart, and encounters with Jesus. *Heart Journey*™ will help many become unstuck and gain forward progress in their pursuit of living wholly!

ANA WERNER
*Founder, President, Eagles Network*
*Author The Seer's Path*

I have had the privilege of knowing Dr. Barbara Lowe, my dear friend and Kingdom co-laborer, for over twenty years. From our early days, it was evident to me that Dr. Barbara possessed a powerful blend of compassion for others, a thirst to understand the inner workings of the human psyche, and a hunger for the deeper elements of God. *Heart Journey*™ addresses the multifaceted aspects of trauma, taking into account the emotional, psychological, and spiritual dimensions that intertwine deep within the human soul. Dr. Barbara draws upon her expertise in psychology and her passion for ministry to guide readers on a transformative path toward wholeness. I am confident, whether you are a person of faith or not, the wisdom shared in these pages will resonate with your deepest longing for healing and restoration. It is both an honor and a privilege to endorse *Heart Journey*™ for anyone seeking to understand the profound impact of trauma upon one's life, while also desiring to embark on a journey of healing. This book is indeed a gift!

DEBORAH KIRBY
*Founder of Joy In The Morning Ministries, Inc.*
*Author, Beyond the Greenhouse*
*Executive Director, Greenleaf Psychological and Support Services*
*Beloved friend and Kingdom co-laborer of Dr. Barbara's Now and Into Eternity*

As a minister, I have spent many years investing in the hearts of women. I have been through many different inner healing ministries, and while this book incorporates many such teachings, Dr. Barbara's *Heart Journey*™ is the most comprehensive inner healing method that I have ever experienced. What distinguishes this book is that it incorporates psychology, biblically-based faith tools, and encounters with Jesus to bring healing to the entire person: body, soul, and spirit. I wholeheartedly believe this is a tool for the body of Christ to be healed, so that we can be whole vessels that can contain the precious oil of the Holy Spirit and not spill it out through all of our wounds and triggers. The resources in this book work even when nothing else has. This book and journal have changed my life, my marriage, and my family. *Heart Journey*™ has healed my heart, brought stability to my soul, and helped my behavior to better reflect my Lord and Savior. This is the case not just for me, but for many friends who have gone on this heart transformation journey with me. It is time for the women of God to arise, repair our vessels, and fill up our oil lamps to be ready for our heavenly bridegroom to come for His glorious bride.

ASHLEY ODVODY
*Mom of Three, Entrepreneur, AACC Certified Mental Health Coach, and Minister*

Dr. Barbara is a true gem, both brilliant and compassionate. She is a lover of God, people, and knowledge. You get to benefit from her years of diligent study and her integration of psychology and ministry experience through her powerful, new book. She is no stranger to trauma, but she is also no stranger to overcoming insurmountable obstacles. Let Dr. Barbara guide you to the healing you are longing for through the *Heart Journey*™ book and journal.

ADRIENNE COOLEY
*Author of the book series Happy ANYWAY, Love ANYWAY, & Believe ANYWAY; Speaker, Senior Co-Pastor of HARVESTMobile.com*

# Disclaimer

I am Dr. Barbara Lowe, Ordained Minister, Licensed Psychologist, Master ART Therapist, Board Certified Life Coach, and Somatic Experiencing Practitioner. I come to you as a Christian Minister, not as a psychologist, as I write solely from an indigenous Christian perspective in this book. In my psychological practice, I always honor and work within the worldviews of my clients. However, as a ministry project, I am presenting this study from a Christian perspective. Of course, there is plenty of room for scientific psychology in a faith-filled Christian life, and I do from time to time refer to standard psychological principles and tools that are available to us all as we heal from trauma.

Please note that all the characters and stories depicted within are entirely fictional, except for Deborah (alias), who consented for me, the author, to share her experiences following the *Heart Journey*™ Method.

This book does not feature any representation of clients from my psychotherapy practice or clinical work.

It is important to emphasize that this book is not intended to be a substitute for therapy. You, as the reader, should not consider yourself as a clinical or coaching client of me, the author, and should always seek guidance from a licensed healthcare provider regarding any health or mental health concerns. This book is intended solely for informational, educational, and Christian edification purposes and should not be used as a replacement for medical or mental health treatment. I have taken care to ensure the book does not contain content that might be overly triggering. However, as this book integrates Christian faith tools, encounters with the Lord, and self-employed psychology tools for inner healing and encounters with Jesus, some content may be triggering. As the reader, you are encouraged to self-monitor and use the skills taught in the first three chapters to self-regulate and reach a solid point of emotional safety. If, at any point, you feel unsafe or need immediate help, you should contact 911.

*The book is dedicated to the hundreds of millions of Christians around the world who face severe persecution, terrorization, imprisonment, and martyrdom due to their faith today.[1]*

*I would like to express my gratitude to ChatGPT, an AI language model developed by OpenAI, for its invaluable help in editing and refining sections of this book. ChatGPT's insightful suggestions and improvements greatly contributed to the final quality of the manuscript.*

# A Note About Language

*Although this book is written for women, it is my sincere hope that any person who would like to engage with this content would feel comfortable doing so.*

# Acknowledgements

I am deeply grateful for the remarkable contributions of Dr. Harold Koenig, Dr. Eric Johnson, Dr. Joshua Knabb, and numerous other pioneers in the field of healing the soul from an indigenous Christian Psychology perspective. Their groundbreaking contributions have paved the way for the profound healing journey within the *Heart Journey*™ framework. In addition, the faith integrative work by Drs. Henry Cloud and John Townsend has been invaluable.

Additionally, I owe a tremendous debt of gratitude to: Dr. Peter Levine, Dr. David Burns, Dr. Marsha Linehan, Dr. Richard Schwartz, Dr. John Bowlby, Dr. Mary Ainsworth, Dr. Stephen Hayes, Dr. Stephen Porges, Drs. John and Julie Gottman, Dr. Sue Johnson, Dr. Bessel Vander Kolk, Dr. Erik Erikson, Dr. Fritz Perls, Dr. Laura Perls, Dr. Daniel Wegner, Dr. Melanie Klein, Dr. Diana Baumrind, Dr. Barbara Fredrickson, Francine Shapiro, Dr. Mark McMinn, Bruce Ecker, Dr. Terrance Real, Dr. Dianne Poole Heller, Dr Heather Gingrich, Dr. Saundra Daulton Smith, Dr. Thomas Chess, and Dr. Alexander Thomas, along with countless other trailblazers who have spearheaded our understanding and healing of the mind, emotions, nervous system, and relationships. Your invaluable insights and advancements have laid many of the foundations for the transformative path of healing found within the *Heart Journey*™. *Heart Journey*™ builds upon your fundamental work.

I extend my gratitude to Dr. William R. Miller and Dr. Harold D. Delaney for their work as editors on Judeo-Christian Perspectives on Psychology: Human Nature, Motivation, and Change, published by the American Psychological Association (APA).[2] Thank you, Drs.

Miller and Delaney, for your efforts in bringing together a work that explores elements of the Christian worldview and psychology that have been relevant for billions of people for millennia. I also express my appreciation to the APA for publishing this valuable contribution.

Thank you to Dr. Thema Bryant, 2023 APA president, for working for "psychology for the people," for acknowledging that your identities and roles as minister and psychologist can coexist, and for your efforts in breaking down prejudice toward the science of psychology in the Christian church. Thank you, "Dr Thema", also for sharing your trauma story freely and publicly.[3]

Furthermore, I would like to express my heartfelt gratitude to my pastor, Bishop Ron Lewis, for his unwavering spiritual guidance and support on all matters, including the birth of my ministry. Your wisdom and counsel have been instrumental in shaping the spiritual foundations regarding the *Heart Journey*™ framework and my ministry efforts. Thank you for your steadfast presence and encouragement throughout this journey. Additionally, I would like to extend my sincere appreciation to Lynette Lewis, the author, speaker, and wife of Bishop Ron Lewis, for her unwavering support and encouragement throughout this process. Your presence, encouragement, and admonishments have been invaluable, and I am grateful for your contributions to the spiritual crossing of the *Heart Journey*™ framework. Moreover, I would like to thank Pastors Reggie and Bomi Roberson for their faithful insights regarding ministry direction. To all of you, thank you for your unwavering support and dedication.

I acknowledge the foundational publications and methodologies created by Dr. Karl Lehman and Dawna DeSilva, as well as in the domain of Christian inner healing.

I would like to extend special appreciations to Dr. Tonya Armstrong, for her sagacious guidance on the ethical considerations pertaining to ministry and psychology throughout the years.

Additionally, the legal advice provided by Steve Shaber, Esq., John Swallow, Former State Attorney General, and Christy Compagnone, Esq., regarding the law pertaining to religious liberty, ministry, and the practice of psychology, has been incredibly beneficial.

Furthermore, I would like to express my appreciation to OpenAI, the developers of ChatGPT, an AI language model, for their invaluable assistance in editing and refining language for significant sections of this book. The insightful suggestions and improvements provided by ChatGPT have significantly enhanced the overall quality of the *Heart Journey*™ book and journal manuscripts. In particular, I would like to extend my gratitude to ChatGPT for its invaluable assistance in refining language, providing editing suggestions, and aiding in the search for relevant Bible sources. ChatGPT's contribution has been instrumental in ensuring the accuracy and authenticity of the *Heart Journey*™ book and journal.

Thank you to Elizabeth Charlé and Kevin White for your invaluable assistance in editing and publishing this work. Your expertise and dedication have greatly contributed to its quality and success.

Thank you to the many content experts in faith, inner healing, and/or psychology who endorsed this work. I deeply appreciate each of you. I am profoundly honored that you took the time to recommend *Heart Journey*™.

Moreover, I want to sincerely thank Ashley Odvody, Ugonna Ukwu, Pastor Verna Brown, Dr. Steve Greene, Dawna De Silva, Nancy Nelson, Elizabeth Johnson, and Deborah Kirby for their incredible support as I developed and wrote *Heart Journey*™.

Lastly, but also primarily, I would like to thank my beloved life-gift, my husband and pastor, Tim Sauve, for all the spiritual formation and encouragement you have lavishly poured into me for decades. You are a large part of who I am becoming, and I thank you with gratitude that is beyond words.

# Table of Contents

# Your *Heart Journey*™

E nvision receiving an inheritance, a house that seems worn and neglected at first glance. Mold, cobwebs, and decay fill its interior. Yet, in this moment, a skilled appraiser arrives and reveals hidden treasures, unique features, and historical architecture. Bursting with enthusiasm, the appraiser proclaims this house as a national treasure, urging you to embark on its restoration. Astonishingly, the appraiser offers to guide and support you throughout the process, free of charge. The only requirement is your time and unwavering commitment. He has graciously pre-paid for all the restoration work you desire, leaving no expense for you to bear.

Dear one, your heart's home is akin to that house, brimming with immense potential and inherent value. The Lord, in His longing to restore you, has already paid the ultimate cost through the precious blood of Jesus. He discerns the profound beauty that lies within, the treasures awaiting discovery beneath the surface. His yearning is to breathe new life into you, mend the broken areas, and unveil the exceptional aspects of your being. With unwavering dedication and unyielding support, He stands beside you as you embark on this transformative journey of restoration. His expertise is unparalleled, for He is the master restorer, and together, you will witness the metamorphosis of your life into a breathtaking masterpiece, filled with His warmth.

Just as in the story of the pearl of great price, where others failed to recognize the greatness of the field, the Master sees the value within you. He sees the pearl of great price that lies within your heart, waiting to be fully revealed and restored. While others may overlook or underestimate your worth, the Master sees your true worth and potential. He invites you to embark on this journey of restoration, where He will lovingly and skillfully restore every aspect of your being.

Beloved, as we set forth on this sacred endeavor of restoring your heart's dwelling, we shall meticulously labor to reinstate its original grandeur. Together, we shall beautify the scars of time and trauma, adorning and dignifying every corner of your soul. We shall explore each hidden nook and cranny, unearthing the treasures of purpose and insight, reminiscent of secret libraries and cozy sanctuaries waiting to be rediscovered. Our mission encompasses the revival of neglected spaces, those affected by the storms of the enemy and abuses of the world.

Moreover, as we engage in this restoration process, you shall experience the gentle and soothing presence of the Lord, permeating every room of your being. Your heart was meticulously fashioned to be a resplendent and tranquil abode, brimming with belonging, satisfaction, and purpose. The time has come to rediscover and embrace your true identity as His beloved, the person you were divinely intended to be. The Lord requests your dedication and commitment, knowing full well that your willingness will catalyze a journey of remarkable transformation.

It is an immeasurable honor for me to join you on this profound journey as we navigate the pages of this book and delve into the transformative *Heart Journey*™ *Journal*. Throughout this expedition, I will stand faithfully by your side, offering unwavering support and guidance in every chapter of this profound journey. In addition, you will have the incredible opportunity to embark on this study with cherished friends or a close-knit small group, fostering a sense of community and shared growth.

As we embark on this sacred path together, I am filled with anticipation for the extraordinary possibilities that await us. The future is brimming with abundant blessings, just waiting to be unveiled. Let us join hands and restore the sanctuary of your heart, igniting its inherent radiance and embracing your divinely appointed purpose that yearns to be fulfilled.

Beloved, the path of restoration may not always be easy, but it is worth every effort. As we set sail on this voyage, let us remember that the restoration of your heart's home is not only for your own benefit, but also for the glory of the Master. As your heart becomes a radiant masterpiece, it will reflect His love, grace, and transformative power to those around you.

With deep gratitude and anticipation, I am honored to accompany you on this sacred journey of restoration. Together, we will witness the extraordinary blessings that await us on this heartfelt expedition. Let us now get to work!

# Introduction to
# *Heart Journey*™ Study Tools

*Heart Journey*™ is a comprehensive book designed to guide us through a transformative process of heart healing and restoration. It provides a roadmap for those seeking emotional healing, inner peace, and a deeper connection with God.

Within the pages of *Heart Journey*™, you will discover a step-by-step process that will move you through stabilizing emotions and the nervous system, to healing unmet needs and traumas, to launching into life's purpose. It addresses various aspects of the heart including past hurts, unmet needs, traumas, nervous system response, parts of self, resentments, fears, shame, and self-judgment. Through engaging exercises and encounters with Jesus, you will be invited to delve into your own story, identify areas of brokenness, and open yourself up to healing encounters with the Lord.

But the journey is not complete with this book alone. The *Heart Journey*™ *Journal* provides a necessary companion resource that will allow you to apply the heart healing process in a more personal and interactive way. The journal is a required complement to the book by providing all the Heartwork exercises and activities that will actually facilitate the heart restoration you seek.

One of the unique features of the *Heart Journey*™ *Journal* is the inclusion of scripted activities that serve as healing meditations with Jesus. These activities are designed to bring you into encounters with Jesus and facilitate a deepening relationship with Him. By engaging with these scripted activities, you can experience transformative moments of connection, healing, and restoration.

To enhance the experience further, both the *Heart Journey*™ book and the *Heart Journey*™ *Journal* offer audio versions of the scripted activities. You can simply activate the QR code provided in the book or journal and submit your best email to access the audio content. This feature allows you to engage in guided Christian meditations and reflections, immersing yourself in the healing presence of Jesus through the power of sound.

Whether you choose to embark on the *Heart Journey*™ individually or as part of a group study, the combination of the book and journal offers a comprehensive and transformative experience. It is an invitation to journey deep into the recesses of the heart, encounter God's healing love, and emerge with a renewed sense of purpose, freedom, confidence, peace, and joy.

*Heart Journey*™ is not just a book or journal; it is a transformative voyage that will empower you to embrace healing, amalgamate with the heart of God, and experience the fullness of purpose for which you were created.

The *Heart Journey*™ study is a powerful resource; however, as noted above, it is important to recognize that reading alone is not enough. To experience true transformation and healing, it is vital to actively engage in the work presented in the *Heart Journey*™ *Journal*.

In the biblical story of the healing at Bethesda, we encounter a man who had been crippled for thirty-eight years. He found himself among many others who waited for healing by the pool. When Jesus saw him, He asked a profound question: "Do you truly long to be well?" This question challenges us to examine our own hearts and desires for healing and restoration.

Similarly, in our journey toward healing and wholeness, Jesus is there to meet us, but we, too, have a part to play. Just as the man had to respond to Jesus' command to "Stand up! Pick up your sleeping mat and walk," we are called to act in our own lives.

By actively participating in the Heartwork exercises in your *Heart Journey*™ *Journal*, you are responding to God's Word and opening yourself up to His healing touch. It is through this intentional engagement that the flow of healing can reach and transform your heart home.

Let Deborah[4] serve as our primary example in this study. She wholeheartedly embraced the work in her *Heart Journey*™ *Journal*, moving from a place where daily heart pain immobilized her, to a life full of purpose and a river of living water flowing through her. Her commitment to the process brought about significant transformation and freedom.

Just like the man at the pool of Bethesda, we may have felt stuck, defeated, and unable to experience the healing we long for. But as we pick up our "mat" of past hurts, resentments, and brokenness, and actively engage in the *Heart Journey*™ process, we position ourselves to encounter the healing power of Jesus.

Similarly, in our journey toward healing and wholeness, Jesus is there to meet us, but we, too, have a part to play. It is important to remember the wisdom shared in James 2:17, which states that "faith without works is dead." Just as the man at the pool of Bethesda had faith that healing was possible, he also had to respond to Jesus' command and take action.

In our own lives, faith is not merely a passive belief, but an active force that requires us to step out in obedience and engage in the work that leads to transformation. Just like the man had to respond to Jesus' command to "Stand up! Pick up your sleeping mat and walk," we are called to take intentional steps forward in our healing journey.

The *Heart Journey*™ *Journal* (sold separately from the study) provides us with the tools and exercises necessary to actively participate in our own healing. It prompts us to reflect, to encounter Jesus's healing in our places of pain, to confront our resentments and fears, to forgive ourselves and others, and to surrender our burdens to God.

By aligning our faith with action, we open ourselves up to the transformative power of God. As we pick up our "mat" of past hurts and brokenness and actively engage in the Heartwork process, we follow Jesus into healing and restoration. It is through our willingness to put in the work that we can experience the miraculous transformation God desires for us.

So, as you embark on this journey of healing and growth, remember that your faith in God's healing power must be accompanied by action. Respond to His invitation, embrace the exercises in the *Heart Journey*™ *Journal*, and trust that as you take intentional steps forward, God will meet you in the process and bring about the healing and wholeness you seek.

I love you, I believe in you, I am with you, and even more, so is He!

Love,
Dr. Barbara

*P.S. For those who have completed your initial journey with the Heart Journey*™ *Study and Journal and desire to dive even deeper into the heart healing process, it is highly recommended to consider purchasing a second journal. Many women have found that going through the Heart Journey*™ *a second time can be a powerful continuation of healing and growth.*

# Notes for Small Group Facilitators

I am so grateful you have responded positively to the calling of facilitating a *Heart Journey*™ small group. I pray that your group experiences many healing encounters through Jesus' powerful love on this journey. To help make the most of this heart restoration process, the following are some suggestions, but please feel free to tailor specific details according to your group's needs.

- This book and journal presents a significant amount of material and includes many activities and opportunities for reflection and discussion. Please feel free to take your time working through the process. I suggest working through the journey with your group at the pace of one chapter every two weeks. Each chapter includes teaching, activities, supporting Scriptures, prayer, and questions for individual reflection and group discussion. To allow time for all of these activities, you will need at least two weekly meetings for each chapter. Then, if you need more time, please feel free to modify the timetable as necessary.

- As you go through this material, please remind the individuals in your group that safety and security is a priority. Healing from emotional wounds can be overwhelming if the process moves too fast; titration and pacing are necessary. If, at any time someone does not feel safe, please encourage them to talk to a professional and not move forward with additional Heartwork until they are ready. Safety is always your priority.

In the rare instance that a life-threatening situation occurs, call 911 immediately.

- During the journey, encourage your group members to make intimate, heart-to-heart connections within your group so they can encourage and pray for one another in between weekly meetings. Facilitate belonging and the felt sense of "every voice matters."

- Those who have been through much trauma may tend to dominate the group with sharing traumas. Keep the sharing balanced among members. Make sure to keep the overall focus more on Jesus rather than the work of the enemy, while encouraging appropriate sharing of the "real." If the group does not meet enough needs for a participant, recommend help from a professional licensed psychotherapist along with the small group. This study is not a substitute for professional mental health care.

- Your role is to facilitate discussion, belonging, support, and prayer, and to share your experience, strength, and hope in Jesus. Never succumb to a pressure to provide counseling, but refer to licensed professional mental health therapists.

# Introduction

Beloved sister, how is your heart? As women, we often find ourselves pouring our energy into others, attending to their needs while unintentionally neglecting our own hearts and minds. But rest assured, God deeply cares about the pain you carry within your heart, and so do I. I wholeheartedly believe that you have been led to this book to receive healing in the innermost places of your pain. This is your time to step into lavish freedom.

I am Dr. Barbara Lowe, Ordained Minister, Licensed Psychologist, Master ART Therapist, Board Certified Life Coach, and Somatic Experiencing Practitioner. I come to you as a Christian Minister, not as a psychologist, as I write solely from an indigenous Christian perspective in this book. In my psychological practice, I always honor and work within the worldviews of my clients. However, as a ministry project, I am presenting this study from solely a Christian perspective.

You are not alone on this journey. Many women have found solace and restoration through the transformative *Heart Journey*™ study. God's healing touch has brought countless women back to a place of wholeness, addressing not only their mental and emotional well-being, but also their spiritual and even physical restoration.

Do you long to be made whole again, to be restored so you can be the incredible and masterful woman God created you to be? This study has been specifically crafted with you in mind. It is designed to nurture that deep longing within your heart, providing a pathway to rediscover a genuine sense of home within yourself—an internal sanctuary of belonging. This study is uniquely designed for the woman who desires to cultivate greater peace, joy, and success in every facet of her life. Whether you are a mother, a wife, navigating the dating scene, pursuing a career, or engaging in ministry, this course is crafted to empower you. Its purpose is to guide you toward a profound sense of wholeness and a genuine feeling of being at home within your own heart and skin.

You may be keenly aware of the pains from your past and the injurious stories written into your childhood story. All of us have experienced traumatic events, unmet needs, and the deceptive lies of the enemy, which have hindered our journey toward wholeness and living out our true purpose. Yet, we were MADE for freedom! Beloved, you are made for freedom, and since you picked up this book, you are demonstrating that you are ready to get free, deep within your heart!

My friend, as I pen these words, I am thinking of you. Through this study, I will be with you through this process of breaking free as you use the tools in the pages to come. I extend a warm invitation for you to discover invaluable skills for cultivating a stable heart, to encounter the transformative healing touch of Jesus, and to step into a life brimming with purpose and wholeness. Rest assured, our beloved Jesus will be your faithful guide throughout this journey, walking alongside you with an unwavering presence—both powerful and tender—guiding you toward a life of freedom and deep fulfillment.

## THE HEART HOME

*Create in me a clean heart, O God,*
*And renew a steadfast spirit within me.*
**Psalm 51:10 (NKJV)**

*Keep your heart with all diligence,*
*For out of it spring the issues of life.*
**Proverbs 4:23 (NKJV)**

The Logos Bible Factbook describes the heart, "the heart is the center, not only of spiritual activity, but of all the operations of human life. 'Heart' and 'soul' are often used interchangeably."[5] Have you ever contemplated how your heart serves as the driving force behind every aspect of your existence? Our hearts, being the seat of our desires and intentions, wield immense influence over our thoughts, words, and actions. It is crucial to consider how God longs to bring wholeness to the home of your heart. Just imagine the incredible impact that a heart made whole can have on every facet of your life. Embracing a restored and thriving heart has the potential to bring forth transformation, joy, and fulfillment beyond measure.

The Scripture reminds us that we are fearfully and wonderfully made, created in His masterful blueprint or image. I often find myself reflecting on the homes of our hearts, envisioning them as captivating, cozy cottages. These dwellings resemble a beautiful, cozy cottage—adorned with shiplap, rugged hardwood floors, inviting brick fireplaces, crisp, white crown molding, and an assortment of textures in every room, emanating warmth and relaxation. However, due to neglect, misuse, vandalism by the enemy, and the storms of life, it has suffered dilapidation over time. The cut flower garden visible from the living room stands ready to produce plentiful yields of flowers to bring the outdoor elements in. However, the once beautiful garden boasts an assortment of stubborn overgrown weeds rather than a colorful display of flowers.

Often, this describes our heart home, does it not? We have frantically focused on the areas requiring immediate attention to keep us functioning, and those past pains and traumas requiring deep mending have been crammed into the basement or an old storage shed. But God wants to restore us to the beauty of what we were intended to be and give us a full sense of treasured belonging.

*I will praise You, for I am fearfully and wonderfully made; Marvelous are your works, And that my soul knows very well.*

**Psalm 139:14 (NKJV)**

Dear friend, have you ever experienced a deep longing for a sense of belonging? Do you find yourself yearning to fit in, to be accepted, and to feel connected, perhaps hoping to alleviate the ache of loneliness? Know that you are not alone in these longings. They are fundamental needs intricately woven into the fabric of your being. You have been uniquely fashioned in the image of a relational God, who has designed you to find fulfillment through belonging, being loved, adored, and embraced in meaningful relationships. These God-given longings of the heart, which you carry within you, are the very needs we aim to address and fulfill throughout this journey. Just as Jesus transformed water into the finest wine at the wedding in Cana (John 2:1-11), we trust that He will pour His abundance into the empty spaces of your heart, satisfying these deep longings and bringing you into a place of fulfillment and joy.

During our upbringing, the Lord's intention was for our parents and the influential figures around us to be strong and safe attachment figures, fostering a sense of internal confidence and security within us. He desired for us to have the assurance that someone has our back and that there is a secure base for us, written into the depths of our hearts. However, without this foundation, we often find ourselves yearning for belonging and safety, sometimes failing to recognize it even when it is present.

Additionally, our nervous system can experience dysregulation, leading to a state of being chronically "on," characterized by heightened anxiety, constant worry, hypervigilance, and a sense of agitation. On the other hand, we may find ourselves trapped in a state of numbness or depression, where we feel emotionally shut down and disconnected from our experiences. Whether we are stuck in an "off" or "on" state, the good news is that we have the power to activate healing and pursue wholeness through the transformative journey of the *Heart Journey*™.

Our heart's home needs rewiring so that we can truly revive deep within. In response to this lack, some of us develop patterns of withdrawing from others and relying solely on ourselves. Some of us reach out to others, but do not feel internally satisfied. But there is hope for healing and restoration. Through this transformative journey, we will explore the pathways of our hearts, allowing the Lord to rewire our understanding of belonging, trust, and reliance on others. Together, guided by the Holy Spirit, we will embark on a process of healing, restoration, and rediscovery of secure attachments.

But first, we want to be sure you feel safe ... this whole study is about restoring safety to your heart, and we want to be safe with ourselves and others. If there are any safety issues, depending on how severe, call 911, go to the hospital, find a psychotherapist, or talk to your doctor. Equivalently, your safety must come before your healing.

Our restoration journey will include rebuilding areas in your life where boundaries were disrupted, meeting unmet needs, and time reversing trauma. And your faithful efforts will enlarge your emotional regulation proficiencies and airlift you into your God-given purpose. Can you sense the immense goodness that is before us, Beloved?

So, my dear one, are you ready to embark on this profound *Heart Journey*™ and discover the remarkable plans that God has in store for you? It's important to acknowledge that this transformative journey may involve navigating emotional pain, but through this process, you will experience a profound metamorphosis. As you engage in this journey, you will be empowered to embrace your true identity as a beautiful, unique, and powerful woman of God. Remember, He already sees the incredible potential within you, and this journey will help you manifest that potential in remarkable ways.

Thank you for allowing me to be with you on this sacred footpath as we enter into the deeper alcoves of the King's abode in search of boundless heart restoration.

Love,

Dr. Barbara

# Heart Journey™ Self-Assessment

*And do not be conformed to this world, but be transformed by the renewing of your mind, that you may prove what is that good and acceptable and perfect will of God.*

**Romans 12:2 (NKJV)**

Using the analogy that your heart is a beautiful, cozy cottage with many rooms, nooks, and crannies, take a few minutes to consider what condition your cottage is in.

Just like in any home remodeling project, it is vital to conduct a comprehensive assessment of the areas in need of repair or improvement before embarking on the restoration process. This entails a meticulous examination of the house, considering both surface-level and structural aspects. Addressing any structural damages requires diligent research to determine the precise tools and supplies needed, ensuring they are readily available. While this initial assessment may appear time-consuming, its significance cannot be overstated, as it paves the way for a seamless renovation. Neglecting proper preparation and using inadequate tools may lead to the temptation of settling for suboptimal solutions, resulting in unnecessary challenges and potential safety hazards.

The journey of reconstructing the heart follows a similar pattern. While on this journey, we will lavishly "stock up" on safety and stability skills to increase our body, soul, and spirit health. We will expand our skills across the domains of healthy thinking, empowering Christian imagery, and self-soothing and positive coping skills. We will also acquire foundational skills in establishing healthy boundaries, which involve discerning what is beneficial and allowing it into our lives while keeping out what is detrimental. We will work on increasing activities that make us thrive, and decreasing those that make us dive. Our initial growth will form a solid foundation for the deeper reconstruction work within our hearts.

In the same way we assess repairs to be made on a home, we must take an objective self-inspection of our heart. To get started, open your *Heart Journey*™ *Journal* and complete the **Assessment, Individual Heartwork - Heart Inspection.**

## SETTING OUR FEET ON THE PATH—HOW TO BEST TAKE THIS JOURNEY

Whether you are going on this journey with a small group or individually, a great deal of information is packed within these pages. As we restore your heart's beauty, you will need time to process the information, delve into the Scripture, and absorb God's message for you. He wants to speak to you and gently guide you on this journey. All our hearts have wounds that need healing. The fragility of your heart varies in accordance with the extent of the trauma you have experienced and your genetic loading regarding trauma resilience. Regardless of your past, Jesus stands ready to walk this path with you, reconstructing your heart with the raw material of His love. And you know Jesus was a master carpenter, right? You are safe in His skillful and adoring hands!

To fully benefit from this study, it is recommended to allocate two weeks for each chapter. This deliberate pace allows for a thorough exploration of the material, which skillfully intertwines a ministry component with a psychological approach. The questions and exercises employed in this study blend ministerial principles with the use of Christianity-infused psychological tools, creating a comprehensive and multifaceted learning experience, facilitating a profound and lasting impact on your life.

As we journey through this process, I encourage you to seize every opportunity to integrate your relationship with Jesus into the study. Allow His presence to permeate your exploration, inviting Him to guide and reveal Himself to you in profound ways. Cultivate a heightened awareness of how the Lord meets you on this transformative journey, recognizing His divine intervention and the ways in which He ministers to your heart.

If you are undertaking this journey as a small group, create opportunities for connections by sharing vulnerably and soulfully and pray for one another. This will nourish you with the sustaining social support you need to rebuild even the most frightening junctions of your heart. If you do not have a small group, consider finding a safe and prayerful friend to go through this study with you.

Exploring past traumas can be a challenging and demanding process, particularly when there has been extensive emotional devastation. It is essential to prioritize your well-being and seek professional support from a licensed psychotherapist if you find yourself regularly overwhelmed during this journey. Additionally, if you reach a point where you realize that delving deeper into the Heartwork feels overwhelming, it is recommended that you focus on the foundational tools provided in the first four chapters. Take the time to strengthen your readiness, and establish a sense of stability before progressing to the next level. Remember, your emotional and mental health should always be a top priority throughout this transformative process.

*He has made everything beautiful in its time...*
**Ecclesiastes 3:11 (NIV)**

Just like the butterfly patiently waits in its cocoon to undergo a remarkable transformation into full flight and glory, Jesus desires to provide the nurturing and care needed for you to transform into your unique blueprint of fullness and beauty. Embrace His guidance and allow yourself to soar to new heights as you undergo this incredible metamorphosis.

Together, let us embrace the adventure and enjoy the journey!

## SPEAKING GOD'S WORD

In Ephesians 6:17, the sword of the Spirit is listed as the Word of God. As the only offensive weapon in God's armor, Scripture serves as a powerful tool to which we have direct and constant access. God loves when we confess His Word out loud and promises us that speaking His Word will accomplish His desires and purpose for our lives.

*The Word of God that I speak from my mouth will not return to Him empty, but will accomplish what He desires and achieve the purpose for which He sent it to me.*

### Isaiah 55:11 (NIV)

*This Book of the Law shall not depart out of my mouth, but I shall meditate on it day and night, that I may observe and do according to all that is written in it. For then the Lord shall make my way prosperous, and then I shall deal wisely and have good success.*

### Joshua 1:8 (AMP)

*I am watching over my word to perform it.*

### Jeremiah 1:12 (ESV)

As you just read in the above Scriptures, God takes the speaking of His words seriously. Beloved, He actually watches over it to ensure it is carried through. The Word of God gives us more than 3,500 promises that cover the gamut of topics we can claim for our daily living. As we study each chapter, it is important to pray the Word of God out loud, especially as it pertains to each section's topic. To facilitate a powerful release of your faith, I have included three Scriptures for each chapter. Beloved, use these as strong offensive weapons to overcome the enemy while on your *Heart Journey*™. Meditate on His living and active Word (Hebrews 4:12), and speak it daily out loud. His Word will change you and your circumstances!

# *Chapter*
## ONE

### Restoring My Heart

*The Spirit of the Sovereign Lord is on me, because the Lord has anointed me to proclaim good news to the poor. He has sent me to bind up the brokenhearted, to proclaim freedom for the captives and release from darkness for the prisoners.*

### Isaiah 61:1 (NIV)

Have you ever found yourself curiously glancing at another woman and wishing your life was more similar to hers? Truth be told, most of us have had this experience. However, if we delve deeper into this longing, we realize that what we truly yearn for is the essence of her heart—that sense of confidence, love, effectiveness, and security. Beloved, God wants to heal your heart home, deep within. He wants you to experience lavish belonging, acceptance, and purpose within your own soul, so you are sumptuously flooded with heartfelt comfort and delicious peace as you pursue the Master's business. But what is the "heart"?

The biblical understanding of the heart encompasses the very core of our existence. It is within the heart that our thoughts, emotions, and will converge, shaping who we are and how we interact with the world around us. Deep within this sacred space, we encounter a myriad of profound feelings: the exhilaration of joy, the weight of sorrow, the warmth of love, and the tenderness of compassion.

Proverbs 4:23 (NIV) encapsulates the significance of the heart beautifully, urging us to prioritize its safeguarding: "Above all else, guard your heart, for everything you do flows from it." This verse underscores the immense impact our heart has on our actions, decisions, and relationships. It serves as a gentle reminder of the vital responsibility we carry in protecting and nurturing our hearts, for they serve as the wellspring from which our lives flow.

Painfully, our hearts are also prone to colossal damage from the culminating abrasions and lacerations of sin, the lies of the enemy, unmet needs, and the ravages of trauma. As a result, we may find ourselves besieged with negative emotions like fear, anxiety, shame, false guilt, self-blame, emotion dysregulation, self-rejection, depression, helplessness, hopelessness, distrust, anger, resentment, and/or bitterness, leading to a shattered sense of peace and contentment in our experiential lives.

Thankfully, God desires to heal every aching nook and cranny of our heart homes and restore us to sustained completeness. In Ezekiel 36:26 (ESV), it is written, "And I will give you a new heart, and a new spirit I will put within you. And I will remove the heart of stone from your flesh and give you a heart of flesh." God wants to replace the limping and aching places in our heart homes with a center that is soft, pliable, whole, and full of His love, belonging, acceptances, and wisdom.

The Greek word for heart, "kardia," used over 160 times in the New Testament, speaks to the depth and complexity of our innermost being, as well as our rich capacity for tender intimacy and profound connection with God. You are built with an endless capability to connect with Him in every deepest abode within your being. You were made to be an endless hub of rivers of living water that nourish every portion of your heart home and luxuriously flow out to others, healing the nations.

Beloved, God is inviting us to present our broken hearts to Him, knowing He will restore and mend us. In Psalm 147:3 (NIV), it is written, "He heals the brokenhearted and binds up their wounds." Together we will experience restoration and become the marvelous building of the Lord, full of Him and equipped to serve the Master more faithfully.

A crucial step in reclaiming the harmony of our heart is recognizing the impact of our past, examining it with honesty, and identifying areas that require healing. It is reassuring to know that God feels our pain (Hebrews 4:15) and longs for our hearts to be whole so we can blast off into our God-given purpose. Areas that are wounded tend to attract debilitating fears and destructive sin patterns that become stumbling blocks to our journey. However, in His immeasurable compassion and love for us, our Father is constantly moved to restore us, not only physically, but also emotionally by meeting our unmet heart needs across our timeline.

He has come to set you free, Beloved (1 John 3:8).

In the following narratives, we will experience the stories of three women who grew up in immensely different childhood environments. Through the experiences of Tonya, Ashley, and Deborah, we will gain insight into how their pasts have shaped the current states of their heart homes.

## TONYA

Excited about going home for the holidays, Tonya is driving home and anticipates being with her relatives. Warm thoughts of her parents, nieces, and nephews envelop her heart. As she prances in, she is embraced. The yummy aroma of turkey and sticky sweet potato casserole wafts throughout the house like waves of baked love. Clanks of fine china give hint to a beautiful table setting where everyone has a place.

Tonya is is brimming with positive emotion as she sits cozied up to her younger sister Ellie, while they watch the kids play on the living room rug where she and Ellie once played. She is bursting with a delicious sense of belonging. Having grown up with this loving family with healthy boundaries where she is seen, heard, accepted, guided, and protected, she has this sense of belonging she carries with her out into everyday life. She experiences an embedded constant whisper to her soul "no matter where you go, no matter what you do, no matter who you are with, we will always have your back."

Even when Tonya is older and most of her childhood nurturers have passed away, she will still feel she has others supporting her—the strong internal sense of "I have backup in life," "I have people there for me," and "I have a felt sense that God will be there for me." That confidence in God came fairly easily to Tonya, as her heart was primed for belonging from her loving family.

## ASHLEY

Ashley, on the other hand, drives home for the holidays with painful flashes interrupting her thought stream of her father's heart-breaking abandonment when she was only eight years old. She then cringes as she remembers how she could hardly tolerate her mom's multiple partners over the years. Driving up to the house, Ashley shivers as she anticipates her mom being intoxicated, joined by her uncle who secretly abused her early in life. Imagine the tension she must feel, thinking about seeing her family. She has some positive feelings, but fear and trepidation overshadow the positive. She feels vacant and terrified all at once.

Throughout her adult life, Ashley has harbored an underlying dread that something awful is always looming, making it challenging for her to trust others. To the external world, she enjoys a successful career, but feels like a fraud due to dark mental and emotional patterns that feel like engulfing black holes of rejection. Ashley will continue to fight a sense of "I do not have backup in life" and feeling like she does not belong anywhere. She feels inescapably trapped by her own negative emotions and an internal sense of chaos around intimate relationships.

## DEBORAH

Within a ministry setting, Deborah[6] worked through the *Heart Journey*™ steps expounded on in this book. She has undergone a profound change through the *Heart Journey*™ Method and has asked for me to share her story here. You will be experiencing segments of her story throughout this transformational study.

Before Deborah's mother, Jeanne, died of colon cancer and prior to Jeanne and Deborah reconciling through a sweet breakthrough in the Lord seven months before Jeanne's passing, Deborah remembers the pain of going home for the holidays. She would strive to feel confident, but would slowly and surely succumb to an anxious and heavy heart.

As Deborah opened the door to her mother's house, Deborah would move to hug Jeanne, and her mother's body would awkwardly tense in resistance as her brow furrowed with repulse. Deborah's life has been marked by the absence of maternal affection and genuine love. Throughout her lifetime, she has experienced a mother who was unable to express love, offer hugs, or engage in any form of meaningful physical touch. Deborah could not remember her mother being comfortable in her presence, unless Jeanne was in the space between tipsy and raging drunk, until the year before Jeanne died. Thankfully,

Jeanne finally yielded to the Lord near the end, and He brought forth a healing in Deborah's heart and in her relationship with her mother.

## YOUR STORY

Beloved, what is your story? Does your story resemble Tonya's or Ashley's? Maybe yours is similar to Deborah's, or maybe you have one that is a combination of all three.

Take some time now to turn to your *Heart Journey™ Journal* Chapter One to reflect and journal on your story. It is healing to write and to share your story. Complete **Individual Heartwork - Your Story.**

## MOVING FORWARD IN HEALING

Observably, no family or scenario is perfect on this earth. We live in a fallen world and were raised by fallen parents by default. Even when we grow up in a healthy home, there can be traumas and abuses that occur outside of the family that break through protective boundaries, leaving us vulnerable and wounded. These experiences can assault us, piercing our safety, giving us a felt sense of damage or injury. Moreover, in every case, we know as Christians that we grow up with an invisible adversary who is always attempting to lie, kill, and destroy our identities and purposes. We have all been impacted; we have all been harmed. God wants you to experience deep and profound overflowing healing in all these areas of soul lesion.

## THE PERFECT PARENT

Thanks be to God, we have continuous access to THE perfect parent in the Lord. He is perfect in love and flawless in boundaries. His extraordinary parenthood is disposed to minister profound healing to your heart.

Even though we have access to this perfect parent, I encountered many women who have experienced childhood traumas and unmet needs, and who thus have a marred relationship with the Lord. They perceive Him through skewed lenses as angry, resentful, or untrustworthy. This is because they have an unhealed attachment lens through which they are seeing and experiencing the Lord. The wounds inflicted by imperfect caregivers can distort our view of God's love, compassion, and faithfulness.

As we go through the healing process, any cloud over your relationship with the Lord will have the opportunity to clear. If you feel distrustful or angry toward God, take comfort that the *Heart Journey* Method™ has helped many women see and experience Jesus afresh, without the patina of the hazy past. Even as the Lord works to mend your heart, some of that cloud, if not all of it, can dissipate, so you can rightly perceive and receive love.

## IT IS OKAY TO NEED!

For many women, acknowledging our needs can be frightening, because we are concerned we will be "too much" or "not enough." As beautiful daughters created by God, each of us has needs.

1. Our hearts need.

2. Our souls need.

3. Our physical bodies need.

Needs are NORMAL! God made you to have them!

We are body, soul, and spirit, and our God-given needs intersect all these domains. When we feel emotions, longings, and needs, neurotransmitters, which are chemical messengers, are released into our bodies, so when we feel, it is not just in our minds, but we experience sensations throughout our physical bodies, our soma. Our spirits long for oneness with God and His love (2 Corinthians 5:1-5). Our souls are an integrative part of us that includes our thinking, our feelings, our will, and our volition or choices. Our souls long for safety, acceptance, love, belonging, connection, healthy boundaries, skillfulness, and purpose.

Furthermore, it is important to acknowledge that as children, our needs were even more extensive than they are now as adults. We were completely dependent on the adults in our lives to meet those needs. As children, we were particularly vulnerable when our essential needs were not met, because we could not take care of ourselves.

Beloved, it is crucial to recognize that the extent to which your needs were met or unmet in the past holds significance for your life today. The recurring patterns of painful relationships and emotional struggles that you find yourself entangled in often stem from crucial needs that went unfulfilled in your earlier years.

So, what do we need in childhood? We will dive deep in on this topic so we can understand ourselves better.

**Safety and Shelter.** Our bodies need safety, and our physical requirements for protection must be met. We also need a home, a place of shelter. The lack of safety and shelter can leave us with a primal felt sense of unmet needs and a dread that "something bad is going to happen."

**Nourishment and Clean Water.** We need healthy meals and clean water for our bodies to function and grow. For the person who has experienced food scarcity, for example, feeling like they are going to have their need for food met can be an area of stress and distrust. I have worked with people who have experienced food scarcity in childhood, and they grow up to be successful and have plenty of food. Yet sometimes they develop eating disorders, hoard food, or have a disordered relationship with food stemming from a lean childhood and fear of lack.

**Protection.** Our bodies need physical protection and to be honored. We need to live in safe homes and neighborhoods, and we need to live free from abuse. When we experience physical abuse or harm, it can leave a lasting traumatic imprint. Moreover, living with a routine threat of being harmed (e.g., by a parent's raging outbursts or living in a high crime area) can have a traumatic impact.

**Secure Attachment.** We require consistent, responsive caregiving by our parents and protective others throughout our childhood. This kind of "good enough parenting" facilitates "secure" brain and emotional organization. Securely attached children usually exhibit healthy self-awareness, eagerness to learn, empathy, resilience to stress, courage to try new things, good problem solving, and strong interpersonal skills. Children who experienced parents who were too often inconsistent, unresponsive, and/or frightening, develop insecure attachment and are less skillful and more anxious, avoidant, or both in relationships. Insecure attachment also lowers self-esteem.

If you grew up in an environment marked by domestic violence or with a caregiver who displayed unpredictability, alternating between moments of love and protection and moments of fear and aggression, it is likely that your attachment system has been significantly impacted. Such experiences can give rise to complications in forming secure attachments. In addition to the example of a parent struggling with substance abuse and its consequent lack of consistency, there are numerous other parental behaviors and experiences that can contribute to insecure attachment in children. These include emotional, physical, or sexual abuse, medical, emotional, or physical neglect, parental absence (intentional or unintentional), frequent criticism, inconsistent parenting, favoritism, a lack of tolerance for negative emotions, and other similar circumstances. These experiences deeply affect a child's sense of safety, trust, and emotional well-being.

**Secure Base.** When we have a secure attachment, we can begin to explore the world with security. Think about toddlers and how they eagerly explore their surroundings, often oblivious to the potential dangers lurking around them. In such instances, it falls upon their parents to vigilantly guide them back to safety and serve as a steadfast and secure base. And when they fall and stub a toe, they quickly hobble back to their secure base. We need our parents to give us space to explore, to be consistent, and to attune to us when we need comfort, especially when we are distraught. A big part of a secure base is having consistent comfort when in duress.

**Autonomy.** Children need a secure base and secure attachment, and as they grow, they also need developmentally appropriate autonomy to be able to explore the world from that secure base. Ultimately, we learn to differentiate from our parents to become a whole adult. Healthy adults are connected with, yet differentiated from others.

**Emotional Safety.** Children need a nurturing environment that prioritizes emotional safety. They need to express both negative and positive valence emotions, and for those sentiments to be accepted. From a biblical perspective, while behaviors can be evaluated as right or wrong, emotions themselves are never deemed wrong. Emotions are part of God's creation, and even He experiences them. In addition, children need a sense of "fit" within their family and primary school and community environments. Children require caregivers who can adapt to their unique needs and personalities, and provide them with a profound sense of belonging. Children also need a generally safe emotional environment, without fear of rejection, harsh words, or inconsistent parenting, where they can expect dependable and responsive caregivers to meet their needs.

**Validation.** As mentioned earlier, it is crucial for children to have their emotions validated. For instance, a parent might respond by saying, "I understand that you're feeling very angry. Your face is red, and your words reflect your anger." It is important to recognize that feelings themselves are not inherently wrong, although our actions in response to them can be evaluated as right or wrong. Therefore, experiencing anger or even being tempted to engage in inappropriate behavior is not inherently wrong. Even when we feel inclined to pout about something, that does not make our feelings invalid. Developing a strong sense of self-compassion toward our emotions is necessary.

While ideally, our parents validated our feelings, there are times when parents may struggle with this aspect. They might respond with statements like, "Why do you feel angry? You shouldn't feel that way." Such responses are unhelpful and fail to meet our need for validation. While it is important to extend forgiveness to our parents, it is equally important to acknowledge our ongoing need for validation of our feelings, which we undoubtedly needed during our upbringing.

If our feelings were not validated during childhood, we may encounter challenges in regulating our emotions as adults. Contrary to some beliefs, validating strong emotions in children actually leads to greater emotional stability, while invalidation has the opposite effect. Therefore, it is essential for our feelings and our very identity to be acknowledged and validated.

**Boundaries.** Children need boundaries, which are rules, expectations, and consequences set by parents or caregivers, to guide their children's behavior and development. Effective boundaries provide children with a sense of security and structure, facilitate the development of principal social and emotional skills, and promote healthy relationships between adults and children. God has boundaries in relationships, and we need boundaries to develop healthy character.

Children need both high warmth and solid boundaries. Children raised by protective others who exemplify high warmth (love) and high structure (boundaries, rules, consistent expectations and consequences) develop into better adjusted adults than those who have high warmth and low structure, high structure and low warmth, or low warmth and low structure.[7] In the example from the "Validation" section above, the parent would say, "I understand that you're feeling very angry. Your face is red, and your words reflect your anger" (warmth). Then the parent would continue with, "Still, you cannot throw your toy doll. Your doll is in time out for three minutes" (structure).

Boundaries serve as a protective framework that allows the good to flourish while keeping the negative influences at bay. Much like the components of a house, such as windows, plumbing, fences, and doors act as healthy boundaries by filtering out harmful elements and preserving what is valuable within. As children develop into adolescence, they need sexuality to be protected, honored, and never abused. We need our parents to help us know and understand boundaries. Over time, we need to develop self-discipline through the examples and structure our parents provide us. Taken together, boundaries make us feel safe and help us develop respect for others and ourselves.

**Regulated Caregivers.** Children develop more optimally when raised by parents or protective others who have regulated nervous systems. When parents are emotionally immature, with emotions and nervous systems bouncing up and down, they have a harder time attuning to the needs of their children. Without consistent caregiving and nurturing, children can grow up feeling like emotional nomads.

Furthermore, it is essential for parents to be free from the inconsistency that addiction can bring, as it can create a dysfunctional and painful environment that stifles authenticity and upsurges the risk for emotional neglect. In families where addiction is present, there are often unspoken rules such as "do not talk, do not trust, do not feel," which can further exacerbate the developmental context. Additionally, family members often are silently yet powerfully forced to inhabit rigid roles such as "addict," "enabler," "hero," "lost child," "scapegoat," or "mascot," which can be detrimental to a child's emotional safety. In addition, it is important to note that where substance abuse is present, all forms of child abuse tend to rise, adding an additional layer of trauma to children who are already struggling with the corrosive rules and roles of a dysfunctional family.

A stable and secure environment, where authenticity is encouraged and rigid role assignments are avoided, can support a child's emotional development and well-being. Parents who have a regulated nervous system and are able to provide emotional attunement to their children can create this type of heart-nourishing environment. By modeling healthy emotional regulation, parents can teach their children how to manage their own emotions and develop the skills they need to navigate the world around them.

**Relational Skills.** God designed us to have a fundamental need for healthy relationships, encompassing safe connections with others, God Himself, and even with ourselves. Cultivating well-functioning relationships requires continuous effort and skillful navigation. Learning how to navigate and create success in relationships with others and ourselves is a central aspect of childhood development. We need to learn how to address conflict, demonstrate empathy, compromise, negotiate, get along with others, navigate disparate social situations, learn how to forgive and set boundaries, and so much more. Without skillfully navigating the realm of relationships, we will inevitably experience a sense of loneliness and defeat, for God intricately designed us to yearn for meaningful connections with others. Navigating relationships skillfully cannot prevent all heartbreak, but it will help us achieve greater levels of relational success and forge the profound connections we are inherently designed to experience.

In addition, have you ever taken a moment to think about the relationship you have with yourself? It is important to remember you are always with yourself, no matter where you go in life. Beloved, nurturing a healthy and positive relationship with yourself requires self-talk, self-forgiveness, self-leadership, self-discipline, self-understanding, and more. Our parents, as competent protectors, can play a crucial role in modeling and teaching us how to navigate relationships with ourselves, filled with kindness and compassion. In addition, we tend to internalize our parents' voices, for better or worse, so while growing up, we need to be handled with validation, gentleness, and empathy.

**Spiritual Development.** We not only need skills in relating to others and ourselves, but we need to be guided toward knowing the Lord and His ways (Deuteronomy 4:9). Introducing children to God is essential for them to believe in Him and develop a personal relationship with Him (Romans 10:14). Children also need to see healthy spirituality lived out, full of grace and truth (John 1:14). Ultimately, children will decide for themselves what they believe, and parents must respect those decisions as well.

**Practical Skills.** Children require practical skills to prepare them for life as healthy and independent adults. It is important they acquire the ability to complete basic tasks such as, taking out the trash, cooking a meal, cleaning the house, maintaining personal hygiene, and caring for a vehicle and home. By learning these skills at a young age, children gain a sense of confidence and independence that will serve them well throughout their lives. These practical skills also contribute to the development of a strong work ethic, self-discipline, and responsibility, which are all essential qualities for success in adulthood. Children need their parents to shoulder the responsibility of teaching and modeling these skills, helping them to become competent and self-sufficient adults.

**Education.** Children need to receive an education that prepares them for career success in their culture. Without a culturally relevant education, children start adulthood behind the starting line of their peers. In the United States, this usually means at least a high school education, but in other cultures, it could mean an apprenticeship or mentorship. We also need opportunities to develop in line with how God made us, according to the blueprint of purpose within us.

**Community.** Children who grow up in safe and non-abusive communities are more likely to thrive and develop into healthy individuals. In contrast, growing up in an environment with high crime or bullying can cause lasting trauma and negatively impact a child's overall well-being.

As children, we rely on our communities to provide a sense of safety and security. When that safety is threatened, it can have lasting effects on our mental and emotional health. For example, exposure to violence or abuse can lead to feelings of fear, anxiety, and helplessness. Bullying can also have a significant impact on a child's sense of self-worth and confidence, leading to issues with self-esteem and social relationships.

Children also need community advocates and protective figures who are watching out for them. These can include parents, teachers, coaches, or other trusted adults who are invested in the well-being of children in the community. By having a support system in place, children can feel more secure and empowered to navigate the challenges they may face in their environment.

## OUR MANY NEEDS

Taken together, God places us in families to shape us, and in childhood, we have certain needs that must be met to become healthy adults. And wow … we have a large number of needs. I wonder how you are feeling right now. It is quite likely that, while reading the above, you encountered areas where your needs were unmet, for our imperfect parents themselves were shaped by imperfect parents. Inherited from generations past, we often carry a legacy of unresolved loss. If you find yourself overwhelmed by these revelations, I encourage you to take a deep breath … inhale the very essence of God's breath and exhale deeply. Remember, dear one, that you are never alone, and help is readily available on your path of healing and restoration.

We can embrace the transformative truth that healing is possible, even in the face of unmet needs and the weight of inherited losses. You have the extraordinary opportunity to partner with God in your personal restoration and experience a remarkable process of "catch-up development." God, the ultimate source of restoration, stands as your unwavering ally. He is unequivocally FOR YOU, not against you, as beautifully affirmed in Romans 8:31. His presence is constantly by your side, offering the precise assistance you require on your journey. Rest assured, He harbors no anger toward you. His love for you is immeasurable, and irrespective of how you currently feel, you are already embraced in His unfailing love and belonging.

*The thief does not come except to steal, and to kill, and to destroy. I have come that they may have life, and that they may have it more abundantly.*

### John 10:10 (NKJV)

Living life abundantly sounds wonderful, does it not? God wants to heal you and pour His blessings over you. Remember … He is THE perfect parent.

## HEALTHY ATTACHMENT

Let us revisit healthy attachment because it is so vital to our emotional and spiritual health. Secure attachment can be likened to a harmonious Venn diagram, where two circles gracefully intersect, symbolizing the connection and closeness between individuals. Yet, within this interconnected space, there is also room for the unique individuality and distinctiveness of each person to thrive. Differentiated means that each individual maintains their own unique identity while still remaining connected and interwoven with the other person. God wants us to become whole people, who are differentiated, but also able to attach to safe others. Healthy attachments allow people to "do life" together, love each other, and support each other. This is where we are going. This is where Jesus is taking us.

It is not healthy for two people to look like two circles, separated completely from each other—this is too differentiated; or if the people in a relationship look like two circles that fully overlap, that is too merged. God desires for us to be integral and interconnected members of His body, harmoniously relating to one another in a manner that promotes health and wholeness (1 Corinthians 12:12-20).

As noted earlier, in the Bible, the heart is understood as the center of a person's innermost being, including their emotions, thoughts, and will. To have a healthy heart home, we need to learn how to have healthy attachments and healthy differentiation, being ourselves and embracing who we are while we relate rightly to others.

*Train up a child in the way he should go,*
*And when he is old he will not depart from it.*

**Proverbs 22:6 (NKJV)**

When childhood attachment needs are not met, we can have a wounded heart home that is either too merged or too differentiated. Beloved, the good news is that the RECONSTRUCTION™ process we will learn in this study will restore these areas by God's power as we faithfully engage in our Heartwork.

## TIME TO RECONSTRUCT!

Now that you have some insight into the condition of all the rooms in your heart, we will look at the heart restoration process, using RECONSTRUCTION™ as an acronym. This overall process can be broken up into three general stages.

## STAGE ONE—SAFETY AND STABILITY

The first step in reconstructing our heart home is to establish safety and stability. In this step, we increase our connection with the Lord, our emotion regulation skills, and our sense of validation. We gain initial skills for nervous system equilibrium that will carry us through the restoration process.

To better understand this, imagine a construction site where a house is being significantly remodeled. The first step is to ensure the safety of the site and assess the inventory of materials needed. This is followed by laying a strong structural foundation. Similarly, before we can embark on reconstructing our heart home, we must ensure the environment is safe and stable. Furthermore, we need to inventory what materials we have and need, and we must gather tools and supplies. Then, we can reconstruct our foundations in safety, well-equipped with the right implements.

## MOVE AT THE PACE OF GRACE

As we embark on the *Heart Journey*™ process, it is essential to remember we do not want our lives to deteriorate within the healing process. We must use the safety and stability skills we are about to learn in the next few chapters to live in an emotionally regulated way, even if we feel pain in the process. We must always stay functional in all key domains of life and even endeavor to enjoy the journey. We have already experienced painful unmet needs and past traumas. All the more, it is important to allow ourselves to experience the gentle healing process of the Master, rather than being driven relentlessly by the harsh voice of the enemy or own, inner critic (Matthew 11:28-30). For example, we never want to just collapse into, "I am just going to suffer and feel this pain, feel this pain, feel this pain, feel this pain, until I cannot function." Rather, we will stay functional and wise through the journey. This means moving at the pace of grace.

Moving at the pace of grace means moving through the process of emotional healing in a way that aligns with God's timing and guidance as we remain in the Window of Tolerance, or a manageable emotional zone. It means learning and faithfully using your stability tools, which you will learn in the next couple chapters. It involves being patient and trusting that God will lead you through the healing process at a pace appropriate for your individual needs and abilities. It also means allowing yourself to experience and process emotions in a healthy and sustainable way, without rushing or avoiding the difficult work of recovery. Additionally, it involves seeking support and guidance from trusted others such as a licensed psychotherapist, your small group, spiritual mentors, and safe friends who can help you navigate the healing process with wisdom and encouragement.

We must live peaceably in our heart home as we go through the *Heart Journey*™ process. Even if we have closed off or ignored certain "rooms" within our heart home for decades, we are still living in this home. Therefore, we must approach this process with care and ensure we maintain a sense of stability and balance throughout. We must achieve mastery with our tools at Stage One before moving into the meaty work of Stage Two.

## STAGE TWO—DECONSTRUCTION AND RESTORATION PROCESS

The next stage of our journey involves heart deconstruction and restoration. First, we identify the unfulfilled needs from your childhood and any traumas that require attention and healing. We will address the detrimental lies that have been sown by the enemy and replace them with wholesome and revitalizing truths. To ease the wounds that have remained from your childhood, we will use encounters with Jesus and a tool named Self-Momming™ to provide the nurturing and love you may have missed. Additionally, unresolved traumas will be carefully addressed and discharged, again using encounters with the Lord and Christ-infused psychological tools. We will also explore areas where boundaries have been violated and actively work toward the restoration of those areas.

At the conclusion of our excavation and rebuilding stage, we will focus on forgiveness. You will learn to forgive both yourself and others, paving the way for newfound depths of delightful freedom and scrumptious peace. Throughout this transformative journey, you will experience comfort and recovery in the presence of the Lord, who will guide and support you every step of the way with His loving hand. His word and presence will change you as we heal the places in your life where the past is still present. As you put in the effort, you will reap the rewards, Beloved.

## STAGE THREE—INTEGRATION AND BECOMING ALL GOD HAS FOR US

The final phase of our journey will prepare us to expand our skills and relaunch into life with newfound confidence, peace, joy, and belonging. Having established a secure heart home, we will be equipped to explore the lavish, purpose-filled life that God has in store for us. We will embrace a new way of living, gaining skills in healthier relationships, and we will make a renewed commitment to spiritual disciplines. As we partner with God in restoration, we will receive double for all that the enemy has stolen through "redo" strategies. Additionally, you will discover and formulate your unique purpose statement and adopt an intentional approach to every aspect of your lives, learning to enjoy a rich and rewarding life of legacy in Him.

So far, we have learned a lot about our needs, some of which likely went unmet in our childhoods. You will turn to *Heart Journey*™ *Journal* and reflect on the questions. You can revisit them later to gauge the progress you and Jesus have made in reconstructing the various areas of your heart.

Take time now to go to your *Heart Journey*™ *Journal* and complete **Individual Heartwork - Your Needs.**

## WE BEGIN

Now that we have explored what the heart truly is and what our journey entails, it is time for us to embark on the next phase of our healing journey—restoring our minds. In the upcoming chapter, we will delve into powerful tools that, when utilized, will produce a delicious sense of stability within our minds. Remember, the next three chapters will prepare us for our deep restoration work within the heart, so delve into Stage One, stability tools, with a whole heart, and faithfully practice your tools daily. Oh, Jesus has so much good for you, dear one!

Turn to **Heart Group Discussion - Time to Share** in your *Heart Journey™ Journal* and complete the activity.

## LET US PRAY.

*Heavenly, Father,*

*We are so grateful that You wish to restore our hearts by bringing us on this restorative journey. We long to be whole, healed, and filled with Your joy, for the joy of the Lord is our strength. As we begin exploring broken rooms of our hearts, may we feel Your agape love and presence.*

*In Jesus' name, Amen.*

# *Chapter*

## TWO

### Restoring My Mind

*"… Even those from afar shall come and build the temple of the Lord.*
*Then you shall know that the Lord of hosts has sent Me to you …"*

**Zechariah 6:15 (NKJV)**

Throughout the Bible, Scripture speaks of rebuilding the temple. Did you know your body is God's temple (1 Corinthians 6:19)? In the same way God rebuilt the physical temple after His people had been in exile from Jerusalem, we are to rebuild our minds and souls back to His healthy blueprint so we can serve Him to the best of our abilities. In this chapter, you will gain many tools you will use in your restoration process. Remember to practice your tools daily.

## THE RECONSTRUCTION™ ACRONYM

As we go through the RECONSTRUCTION™ acronym, naturally we will start with the letter "R." If you will permit (this may seem a little peculiar), we will go right into another acronym with the "R" of RECONSTRUCTION™ standing for RESOURCE™. Many of our Stage One tools that will prepare us for the deeper work will come through our RESOURCE™ tools.

## RESOURCE™

You are about to learn a range of valuable *Heart Journey*™ RESOURCE™ skills that can bring stability to your mind, emotions, nervous system, and relationships, allowing you to experience a sense of being deliciously grounded. Every tool will be embedded in a Christian framework. Our RESOURCE™ skills will give us more mental and emotional equilibrium and help us stay in what is called the Window of Tolerance.

## WINDOW OF TOLERANCE

We function at our best and heal more effectively when we can maintain our nervous system within a specific range called the Window of Tolerance, which is neither too high nor too low. This range, also known as the resilient zone, is where our nervous system functions smoothly, and we feel mentally, emotionally, and bodily in control. When we are triggered, we can become hyper-aroused (too high) or hypo-aroused (too low), which can impact our ability to function optimally in mind, emotions, and body. Hyperarousal occurs when we are too close to the fight or flight zone, resulting in experiences of anger, agitation, anxiety, and a sense of not being in control of our reactions. When we function out of the more primal parts of our brain, such as the limbic system and cerebellum, our brain is concerned with survival rather than with functioning wisely. In contrast, hypo-arousal can lead to depression, numbness, dissociation, and exhaustion. In states of hypo- and hyper-arousal, when we are in survival mode, our access to the neocortex, the region responsible for higher-level processing, becomes limited. Beloved, we do not heal while in survival mode.

Hence, it is vital to cultivate self-awareness, self-monitoring, and self-leadership skills to recognize when we are nearing the edge of the Window of Tolerance and utilize tools to restore balance. As we work on deeper issues of the heart, we must remain in a manageable nervous system zone, even if we experience pain. By staying within the Window of Tolerance, we can function at our best and ensure that our brains and bodies are operating effectively.

Therefore, Beloved, we want to master our RESOURCE™ skills so we can prevent or recover from moving out of the Window of Tolerance. With this mastery, we can more effectively move into the deeper heart healing exercises that begin in Chapter Five. Again, I cannot overstate the essentiality of learning, practicing, and mastering RESOURCE™ tools. Our King and role model, Jesus, walked in unbroken peace and demonstrated the fruit of self-control consistently even through deep trials. Let us commit to follow His example.

Dear one, can you sense the hope that lies before us? As you develop your RESOURCE™ skills, you will find yourself moving toward a state of delicious stability. The first letter of RESOURCE™ is "R," which represents the skill of reframing. Learning how to reframe is the initial step toward stabilizing and enhancing safety in our lives.

## REFRAME

Reframing has origins in Scripture. For example, Romans 12:2 (NIV) says, "do not conform to the pattern of this world, but be transformed by the renewing of your mind." Reframing involves cognitive restructuring and was expounded through the work of American psychiatrist, Aaron Beck. A metaphor might help us here. Think of an art print. Now imagine that print framed with a homely, scuffed up frame. How does it look and feel? Next, imagine that same print framed with an elegant frame. How does it look and feel now? The frame changes everything!

Our thoughts are similar in that they frame our interpretations of life situations with "spin." As we go through experiences, we interpret life via our thoughts, and those thoughts shape what we feel, believe, and do. Like the frame metaphor above, our perceptions of what happens to us often shape our inner world more than the events themselves. They shade how we see the world.

We talk to ourselves all the time, but our thoughts and perceptions are not always helpful. Many of our thoughts are unhelpful, even categorically destructive. Often, our thinking falls into themes or scripts. Neurons that fire together, wire together. Like a river that follows the same path day after day, so are our thoughts. As examples of typical scripts, we might magnify situations that are negative, shrink situations that are positive, or engage in "mind reading" (i.e., thinking we know what others are thinking). We think we know what others are going to say, what they are going to feel, or what they are thinking about us. Sometimes, we can have an overly critical mind toward ourselves, manifesting in a pervasive and nagging felt sense that "I am not good enough" or "I am too much." Over time, these destructive scripts become stronger through repetitive thinking. They feel like weights on our minds, dragging us down. But we can change all that!

## REFRAME BY INVENTORYING YOUR THINKING

In your Heartwork, you will work on "Inventorying Your Thinking." We will inventory our thoughts on a daily basis, looking for scripts that are not helpful, energy draining, and peace destroying. Subsequently, we will use truth to consume and destroy those painful mental fortresses. God wants your mind free from the entangling cobwebs the enemy has woven into your neural pathways. It is time to experience the relief of right, godly thinking (James 3:17).

For instance, let us revisit our friend Deborah from Chapter One, who grappled with deep-seated fears of rejection and abandonment, particularly in her relationships with women, especially those in positions of authority. This thinking was ingrained in her dysfunctional relationship with her mother. Deborah learned to identify her negative thoughts and perceptions, (e.g., mind reading: "my supervisor likes the other employees more than me") and volitionally reformulate every thought into a truthful script. This process of frisking her thoughts for misrepresentations and replacing the enemy's deceits with the soothing balm of genuine truth developed more stability in her mind and her emotions.

In psychology, "terminal uniqueness" refers to the belief or feeling that one's problems or situation are completely unique and cannot be understood or helped by others, which is a common struggle for most of us. We tend to judge ourselves harshly, feeling exceptionally dissimilar from others and comparing the worst version of ourselves to the highly edited presentations of others. However, the truth is we all have internal struggles and need to clean up our minds from ingrained, automatic scripts of rejection, inadequacy, shame, and fear.

Automatic thoughts are those we have spontaneously in response to a situation or trigger, and they are often outside of our direct awareness. However, we can develop awareness and change these thoughts. Some common automatic thoughts include:

1. "I am going to be rejected."

2. "I am not good enough."

3. "I am too much."

4. "I am not safe."

5. "I am guilty; it is all my fault."

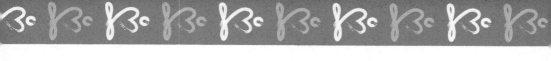

6. "I am not worthy of love."

7. "I cannot trust anyone."

8. "I am defective."

Beloved, it is crucial to become aware of these unhelpful thoughts that contribute to your pain and instability. It is time to allow God to reign over your mind with His higher thoughts (Isaiah 55:9) and begin to speak to yourself as you would to your dearest friend. Remember that Jesus resides within you and desires you to treat yourself with kindness and compassion.

As we take inventory of our thoughts, we may notice that they often fall into one of three categories: defectiveness, safety, or trust. The defectiveness category includes unhelpful thoughts such as "I am damaged" or "I am not good enough." The safety category includes thoughts like "I am not safe," while the trust category includes thoughts like "I cannot trust anyone," including ourselves, others, and even God.

Beloved, it is time to take an inventory of your thoughts and reframe them into truthful assertions. We will also commit to searching for and applying Scriptures that contradict any harmful thoughts. We will replace lies with God's truth. We know that the Word of God is powerful and active, separating soul and spirit (Hebrews 4:12), and speaking His truths demolishes the works of the enemy in our lives (Matthew 4:4).

*For the Word of God is living and powerful, and sharper than any two-edged sword, piercing even to the division of soul and spirit, and of joints and marrow, and is a discerner of the thoughts and intents of the heart.*

### Hebrews 4:12 (NKJV)

Friend, it is important to recognize the immense power you possess over your thoughts. Although you cannot control the thoughts that arise in your mind, you have the ability to decide whether to allow them to linger. Keep in mind that meditating on truth is a potent tool, and if you cannot find a suitable Scripture to dwell on, you can instead focus on thoughts that align with biblical principles. By consciously directing your thoughts toward what is true and in accordance with God's Word, you can actively shape and influence your thinking patterns.

Moreover, it is of utmost importance to extend the same kindness and compassion toward ourselves as we would to others. Often, we find ourselves being much harsher and critical toward ourselves than we would ever be toward our worst enemy, and this harmful self-talk must be transformed. Let us begin to relate to ourselves with the same gentleness, understanding, and grace that we would offer to our dearest friend. When we embrace ourselves with God's boundless love, including self-love, that love will emanate from within us, blessing those around us like the fragrant aroma of the sweetest incense.

As you turn to your *Heart Journey*™ *Journal* to Chapter Two and complete your **Inventory Your Thinking Heartwork**, let lies that have bogged you down like wet blankets slip off as you receive the truth of God's Word that will heal your soul and lighten your load. Then, we will discover another formidable reframe tool.

I am so proud of you for turning your thinking around! Keep using your Inventory Your Thinking tool daily. Now we turn to our second reframing tool, Mind Mansion™.

## REFRAME THROUGH THE MIND MANSION™ TOOL

Another Reframing imaging tool is my Mind Mansion™, which is based on positive psychology and Philippians 4:8.

> *Finally, brethren, whatever things are true, whatever things are noble, whatever things are just, whatever things are pure, whatever things are lovely, whatever things are of good report, if there is any virtue and if there is anything praiseworthy—meditate on these things.*

### Philippians 4:8 (NKJV)

Jesus skillfully employed the power of holy imagination to captivate the hearts and minds of His listeners. Through the use of parables, He invited them to engage their imagination and enter into vivid mental images that conveyed profound spiritual truths. By appealing to their imagination, Jesus created an experiential learning environment, enabling His teachings to deeply resonate within their souls. He recognized the transformative potential of holy imagination, encouraging His followers to embrace the beauty of divine imagery and envision a reality that transcended the limitations of their physical circumstances. Similarly, we can use our holy imagination to reframe our thinking into positive, God-centered neuropathways rather than dwell in familiar negative bogs.

In John 14:2, Jesus said that the Father's house has many rooms. Have you ever considered that your mind has many quarters? Jesus lives inside of you and wants you to use your mind to enter into rooms of joy, peace, patience, kindness, wisdom, gentleness, and the like. Father God created your imagination, not to be used to paint menacing scenes through worry and fear, but for the true, good, pure, and lovely.

In this mindset, I ask you to consider visualizing your mind as a vast and expansive mansion, containing an abundance of rooms. This mansion is unlike any other on Earth, towering high, stretching out in all directions, and plunging deep below the surface and high into the heavens, with millions, if not billions, of rooms at your disposal. You have access to each and every one of them.

In each room lies a door on the ceiling, the floor, and every wall, affording you the freedom to exit any room at any time. There are no locked doors, and you can teleport to different rooms as desired.

In my experience, it is common for women to find ourselves habitually spending extensive time in certain dingy and dark rooms of our mental mansion. These rooms can be found in the basement areas, filled with cobwebs and ominously murky atmospheres of anxiety, worry, and shame. Despite the pain we experience in these rooms, we keep returning here, day after day. It is almost as if we are drawn to these frightening areas, possibly due to their familiarity. However, it is important to recognize that we have the power to choose which rooms we spend time in and can explore the vast and expansive mansion of our minds with Jesus.

It is time to recognize you have the ability to explore any room within your mansion and ponder countless true, noble, just, pure, lovely, and good possibilities. Jesus is calling you out of the muck and the mud of your mental habits. What do you want to think about? Maybe you want to go to the Bahamas for sixty seconds, or maybe you want to go back to a pleasant memory from your childhood? Perhaps you want to remember your favorite childbirth memory or the day you became a Christian? The possibilities are endless!

Moreover, you can experience real encounters with Jesus in your Mind Mansion™. Remember, He is in you, and you are seated in heavenly places in Him (Ephesians 2:6; 1 John 4:12-13). Because He is in you and you are in Him, you can invite Jesus into the rooms of your Mind Mansion™. You can have a tea party with Jesus or go to a baseball game with Him, anywhere you want, all within your own Mind Mansion™. You can also bring Jesus into the dark and dingy rooms in your Mind Mansion™ and redecorate.

Our friend, Deborah minored in French, and she loves French culture. As she engages with the Mind Mansion™ tool, she walks the scenic streets of Paris, enjoying pastries and heading toward street artists painting the Seine River. She invites Jesus into her French experience, and they make a day of it. He is so nurturing and attentive, and she drinks Him in as a secure attachment figure. After a lovely afternoon, Deborah invites Jesus to redecorate the basement (the room with the thoughts of rejection) with a lovely French-themed motif.

Now it is your turn. In what rooms do you want to spend time within your Mind Mansion™? How do you want to interact with

Jesus in Your Mind Mansion™? What rooms do you and He want to redecorate?

As you turn to your *Heart Journey*™ *Journal* and work on **your Mind Mansion™ Heartwork,** use your holy imagination to bring forth the fruit of love, joy, and peace into your mind. Choose rooms that will regulate you and welcome Jesus into every room with you.

Go to the **Mind Mansion™ Activity** in Chapter Two of your *Heart Journey*™ *Journal.*

Use this QR code to access audible versions of activities.

After you complete your **Individual Heartwork - Mind Mansion™ Activity,** take time to complete your list of **Individual Heartwork - Pleasant Thoughts** in Your *Heart Journey*™ *Journal.*

## REFRAME THROUGH DAILY JOURNAL PRACTICE

Journaling daily is a great way to practice your reframing tools, such as Inventory Your Thinking and Mind Mansion™. By reflecting on your old mental scripts and writing out new thoughts using Scriptures as medicine (Psalm 107:20), you can turn negative habitual thinking around. At the end of the day, you can review how well you were able to do this and how effective it was in lifting your mood as your thoughts become more merged with God's way of thinking.

For instance, if you said something in a meeting that nobody commented on, and you start to "beat yourself up" over it, you can use your journal to reframe the situation. Ask yourself, "What would my best friend say about that statement and thought?" Most likely, your best friend would say it was a good statement and express pride in you for saying it. You can also ask yourself, "What does God say about me?" and paint your mind with a helpful Scripture or ask God directly what He says about you.

Journaling also helps solidify positive experiences using the Mind Mansion™ tool. After an emotionally trying day, use your imagination (Philippians 4:8) to go into your Mind Mansion™ with Jesus and leave your worries behind. Have fun with Jesus and play, as fun and play are essential for good mental health. Your imagination has no bounds, and no good thing is off-limits when having fun with Jesus in your Mind Mansion™.

Let us quench the flames of worry by redirecting our focus to Jesus through our holy imaginations. Trying to stop a thought by simply telling ourselves not to think it rarely works. For instance, if I told you not to think of a brown bear, what would you think of? A brown bear, of course! So, it is more useful to intentionally think about something else, such as meditating on Jesus. As we fix our eyes on Him, the worries of this world will fade away. Women tend to ruminate on worried thoughts, which cheat us of joy and peace. Worry is the opposite of faith and is detrimental to our mental health. We need to stop giving in to the obsessive temptation to worry and start mediating on the abundant love and goodness of God.

> *Be anxious for nothing, but in everything by prayer and supplication, with thanksgiving, let your requests be made known to God; and the peace of God, which surpasses all understanding, will guard your hearts and minds through Christ Jesus.*
>
> **Philippians 4:6-7 (NKJV)**

Next, we will learn more uses for our holy imagination to reach emotional equilibrium. I am giddy to introduce you to Enrich with Imagery tools!

## ENRICH WITH IMAGERY

We are focusing on foundational RESOURCE™ skills, and the letter "E" stands for "Enrich with Imagery." This skill is particularly important for Stage One, Safety and Stability. Many people find visual imagery effective for regulation; however, if visual imagery is not impactful in soothing your emotions, consider tactile or auditory imagery as you use your holy imagination.

## ENRICH WITH POSITIVE MEMORIES

With Enriching with Positive Memories, our goal is to find five to ten highly positive, unadulterated positive memories to bring to mind when needed to self-soothe. To begin enriching with imagery, focus on formative positive memories that evoke a robust sense of keen emotional safety, confidence, and belonging. It is important to keep in mind that our goal in this initial stage is to cultivate a greater sense of security and stability, which will enable us to navigate difficult experiences with greater ease while maintaining our overall well-being and functioning. Developing this skill will better equip us to handle whatever challenges we may encounter and stay within the Window of Tolerance.

Find images that are as positive or empowering as possible, and are not corroded by negative "feeling" elements. Nonetheless, it is important to note that sometimes when we attempt to recall a positive emotional memory, other traumatic or difficult memories can attempt to interfere. This is a common experience many people face.

To begin the exercise, turn to your *Heart Journey*™ *Journal*. Take some time to reflect and identify a strong, positive, emotional memory that evokes a sense of safety and comfort.

Complete the **Enrich with Positive Memories Activity** and the **Uncoupling Activity.**

Use this QR code to access audible versions of activities.

## UNCOUPLING AND POSITIVE MEMORIES

Incorporating the above uncoupling tool can help us disentangle negative emotions from positive memories. This process enables us to harness positive memories as a source of comfort and safety, ultimately allowing us to experience joy and positive emotions, which God desires for us. We are not denying our negative emotions, but containing them so we can experience the benefits of positive memories.

According to Barbara Fredrickson's research, we thrive when we have three positive emotions for every one negative emotion. It is God's will for us to flourish and enjoy our lives. While suffering in obedience is part of our walk with Christ, we should not settle for perpetual suffering due to being wounded, as Jesus Himself stated that He came to give us abundant life (John 10:10).

As an example of uncoupling, Deborah's grandparents were very important to her, and her grandmother's cookie jar represented love and warmth. Unfortunately, Deborah's grandparents have passed away, and the memory of them can often be tinged with sadness. If Deborah finds that thinking about the cookie jar brings up feelings of grief or loss, she may want to try to uncouple those negative emotions from the positive memory.

The goal here is to use the imagery of the positive memory as a tool to create a sense of love, comfort, validation, and belonging for ourselves. Belonging refers to the feeling of being accepted, valued, and included, and validation refers to our thoughts, feelings, or experiences being heard, recognized, accepted, and understood.

By pinpointing an object in the room that embodies the negative emotions linked to the positive memory, we can extricate the positive from the negative, and bask in the positivity of the memory without being held captive by the negative emotions. At times, we become so accustomed to feeling down that negative emotions consume us, giving us no respite. Uncoupling helps us find relief.

Deborah could practice uncoupling by associating the positive memory of her grandparents with a picture and the negative emotions with a nearby vase. This would allow her to experience both emotions separately, and thus she can fully appreciate the warmth and comfort the positive memory brings without being stuck in the distress of negative emotions.

Processing grief and acknowledging the full range of our emotions, rather than suppressing them, is important. However, for the purpose of this activity, we will focus on identifying positive memories that bring us a sense of belonging, comfort, and happiness. These could be memories of a beloved beach house, a special connection to the mountains, or any other place that elicits positive emotions and feelings of safety. You may have already formed healing relationships with certain places over time. Think of your childhood treehouse or a transformative mission trip to Tanzania.

Take a moment to go to your *Heart Journey*™ *Journal*, reflect, and make a list of these positive memories as assets in your journal, adding them to your Pleasant Thoughts list. This list will be helpful in replacing negative thoughts and memories with positive ones, allowing you to tap into a sense of safety and comfort during difficult times.

## ENRICH WITH SAFE PLACE IMAGERY

Another exercise for enriching with imagery is known as Safe Place. This exercise has been effective in helping individuals achieve emotional safety and regulation of their nervous system and is found in many therapy modalities. However, before the science of psychology came into existence, the Lord was already using safe place principles in the Scripture. Think about Psalm 23. Why do we love this psalm so much? I believe it is because the imagery washes over us with safety, love, acceptance, and protection.

Here, we will again use our holy imaginations according to Philippians 4:8. We will use our imagination to develop a place we can go to with Jesus in our minds that is unreservedly and entirely safe. This is our special space we can go to for nervous system regulation. It will be important to put items you love to see, touch, hear, smell, and even taste in this safe place with Jesus. Perhaps you can even ask Jesus if He has ideas on how to furnish and decorate your safe place. Your safe place can be as big as you want, and it can be an inside space, an outside space, or both. There are no limits as long as we stay in the realm of what God would consider good according to his word.

Take some time to go to your *Heart Journey*™ *Journal* and go through the **Safe Place Activity** now.

Use this QR code to access audible versions of activities.

If you found the Safe Place exercise helpful, it is a good idea to make it a part of your daily routine to promote feelings of calm and safety. When you connect with God's Spirit in that space, you can cultivate a deeper sense of everlasting intimacy, peace and security. The more you set your heart gaze on Him, the stronger your heart and the more whole it becomes. It is worth noting that some people with artistic skills choose to enhance their Safe Place experience by painting or drawing their special space. Creating a visual representation of your safe place can further enrich the experience.

We have one more Enriched with Imagery activity. As we use our holy imagination again, prepare to have an encounter with our Jesus.

## ENRICH WITH EYES OF JESUS™

Have you ever considered why eye contact is difficult for many? Eye contact is intensely personal. In fact, the Bible says the eye is the window to the soul (Matthew 6:22-23). Through eye contact, we can soften into connection, but the converse is also true. At times, we have received the brunt of anger and hate that has come through a mean-spirited gaze.

As I write this, I am curious ... what is your experience with eye contact? Do you feel comfortable holding a gaze with others? With whom are you comfortable holding eye contact? What was your experience of eye contact in childhood? As we reflect on the significance of eye contact in fostering social connections, we are reminded of our innate and God-given need for healthy relationships. However, we must also acknowledge that eye contact can sometimes lead to negative experiences such as unwanted lust, anger, rejection, hatred, and other hurtful intentions. In addition, the lack of eye contact can represent neglect, being over-looked, or being ignored.

From this brief discussion, we can understand that we have all received relational nourishment and attachment as well as pain and abuse through eye contact. In addition, because we innately know that through our eye contact, others gain access to a window to our soul, we can shy away from eye contact due to our own negative viewpoint of ourselves.

Jesus desires to bring you healing through His gaze. He longs for us to look into His eyes and receive the overflowing and boundless love that pours out from the depths of His soul. Jesus desires for you to experience a sense of belonging with Him that exceeds what you could ever imagine or dream.

Now take out your *Heart Journey*™ *Journal* and complete the **Eyes of Jesus**™ **Activity**. Allow yourself to be enveloped in His love, knowing that as His love heals your heart, you will receive more and more over time, just as Jesus said in Matthew 13:12.

Use this QR code to access audible versions of activities.

Now take out your *Heart Journey*™ *Journal* once more and complete **Individual Heartwork - Enrich with Imagery**.

## STRUCTURE YOUR LIFE

As we continue with RESOURCE™, we will look at the "S" (in the RESOURCE™ acronym), which stands for structuring our lives.

Up until this point in the RESOURCE™ acronym, we have studied and practiced Reframe, Enrich with Imagery, and now Structure Your Life. Again, these tools are essential in establishing a foundation of safety and stability before we plunge into the deeper heart repairs.

Structure Your Life is a life balance tool that places emphasis on the significance of equilibrium. With this tool, we will assess how we are spending our time and energy and look for where God might want to prune. John 15:2 says, He prunes all who are in Him to make us more fruitful. Are you willing for some pruning, Beloved, if it will extend your energy and vitality?

## HOMEOSTASIS

All living beings require and seek homeostasis or equilibrium, including humans. The Lord created us for balance. Unfortunately, due to our wonderful, but driven higher cortex, we can obstruct our path and press ourselves too hard in some areas while neglecting ourselves in others. Adequate sleep, proper nutrition, exercise, work, play, time with Jesus, and healthy relationships are all fundamental in establishing a well-balanced life. Attaining this balance is imperative throughout the healing process, as it enables greater stability and resilience. Dearest one, it is essential to remember, you must treat yourself with the same kindness and compassion you would show a treasured friend.

## STRUCTURE YOUR LIFE: SELF-CARE

As a clan of women, some of us can admit to employing busyness while neglecting our inner realities. We often busy ourselves with rallying around others while disregarding what is truly required for a balanced life. We also may turn to food or other addictions as a way of escaping life's stressors rather than rightly squaring our lives. In order to mend, it is essential to maintain a sense of balance. Self-care is not selfish, but is an essential component of our overall well-being and is necessary for us to function optimally. The Bible teaches us to love our neighbors as ourselves, which implies we should also love and care for ourselves. Jesus Himself took time to rest and recharge, setting an example for us to follow.

## STRUCTURE YOUR LIFE: LIFE EDIT

The Bible speaks often of "metanoia" which means changing our mind and behaviors to align with truth and with God (e.g., 2 Corinthians 7:10). It is time to make some changes to bring balance. Otherwise, we will have little bandwidth for healing.

To achieve balance, it is beneficial to identify the activities and individuals that either energize or deplete us. Activities that provide us with energy are often those for which God has granted us grace (Zechariah 4:6). Conversely, those that drain us may be what are referred to as "dead works" in the Bible. Dead works involve engaging in activities we were either never meant to do, or engaging in activities we were previously called to do, but have now been called out of. We should strive to limit the time we spend on energy-draining activities while staying true to our inner compass, the Holy Spirit, with how we spend our time (Galatians 5:16-17).

Have you ever decluttered your closet and sifted through your wardrobe, separating clothes that no longer fit your style? Perhaps you sorted them into baskets labeled "give away" or "throw away." In the same way, we will edit our life activities. Some activities may no longer suit us, while others may never have been a good fit to begin with (just like that dress we bought but never wore). Like the closet analogy, to free ourselves from certain activities, we may need to "give them away" or delegate the responsibility to someone else.

Evaluating the percentage of time we devote to work, family, hobbies, socializing, and fellowship with believers and God, sleep, and movement are also important in determining our lives' balance. We must assess how we spend our time to make any necessary changes. Seeking feedback from someone close to us may also provide valuable insight, especially when we are overly critical of ourselves! Consider asking a friend, "Do you see an activity in my life for which I clearly do not have grace?"

When thinking about editing our lives, we also must think about our values. What do you value most? Look at how you spend your time and look at your values. Is there an overlap? What do you need to change to make sure your time allocation is concordant with your values?

Moreover, whether we value rest or not, we must learn to respect the need for rest that God has placed within us. As we structure our lives, we must seek balance, which includes self-care and spirit-care. Our God created the Sabbath for rest and modeled this practice for us to care for ourselves. We should aim for one-seventh of our lives to be devoted to Sabbath rest.

## STRUCTURE YOUR LIFE: SEVEN TYPES OF REST

Dr. Saundra Dalton-Smith, a medical doctor, author, and friend of mine has identified several types of rest crucial for establishing proper life rhythms: physical, mental, emotional, social, sensory, creative, and spiritual rest.[8]

Physical rest involves giving our bodies adequate sleep, exercise, and relaxation time. Mental rest involves quieting the mind and minimizing mental stimulation. Emotional rest is achieved by processing and releasing emotions in a healthy way. Social rest involves setting boundaries and taking time for meaningful connection with loved ones. Sensory rest involves minimizing exposure to sensory stimulation, such as noise and screens. Creative rest involves engaging in activities that promote creativity and allow us to express ourselves. Spiritual rest involves connecting with Jesus and engaging in spiritual disciplines.

Rest is essential for maintaining physical, emotional, and mental health, as well as for preventing burnout and promoting overall well-being. Incorporating intentional rest into our daily routines can lead to greater productivity, creativity, and fulfillment. Beloved, where are you finding rest for your soul? Like the law of gravity, the law of rest is not optional. What goes up must come down to rest.

*Come to Me, all who are weary and heavily burdened [by religious rituals that provide no peace], and I will give you rest [refreshing your souls with salvation]. Take My yoke upon you and learn from Me [following Me as My disciple], for I am gentle and humble in heart, and you will find rest (renewal, blessed quiet) for your souls. For My yoke is easy [to bear] and My burden is light."*

## Matthew 11:28-30 (AMP)

Rest is imperative, as is relationship nourishment. We should also assess the relationships in our lives and determine whether they are energy-giving or energy-draining. Relationships that are God-centered and life-giving create a sense of flow and fill our hearts. We should spend thoughtful time nurturing life-giving relationships while considering pruning back life-draining relationships, especially during the healing process while our energy is needed for restoration.

As you work through your Heartwork, pray over what God might have you edit out of your life, and obey Him. There is no quicker way to the finish line of wholeness than obedience. In addition, as you inventory your values, prayerfully ask the Lord if He wants to edit your values. Seek Him for alignment with Him and His values. In addition, we will complete boundary work in future chapters, but for now, consider spending less time with energy-draining people where you can, and more time with energy-giving people. As you go through the healing process, you will particularly need to conserve energy for mending.

Turn now to your **Individual Heartwork - Enrich with Imagery, - Structure Your Life, and - Staying in My Window,** as well as **Heart Group Discussion - Time to Share** in your *Heart Journey*™ *Journal* and complete the activities.

Beloved, I am so proud of you. We will press on together, and even as I write these words, I see His brilliant light of belonging shining upon you and into you. He is lifting up your countenance and expressing His deep love and admiration for you, even right now. Know that you are deeply loved.

In the next chapter, we will resume our work through the RESOURCE™ acronym and continue moving forward with our stability work. After completing the next chapter, you will have a strong and sturdy tool belt full of skills for safety and stability. You are doing great, Beloved. Keep pressing on and practice your RESOURCE™ tools daily.

*Beloved, I pray that you may prosper in all things and be in health, just as your soul prospers.*

**3 John 1:2 (NKJV)**

## LET US PRAY.

*Heavenly Father,*

*Again, we are so grateful that You have brought us on this healing journey, especially with sisters in Christ who can help bare our burdens. We pray You will be with each one studying this lesson as she works toward renovating the innermost chambers of her heart.*

*In Jesus' name, Amen.*

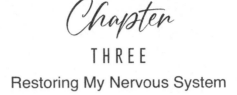

*Chapter*

# THREE

## Restoring My Nervous System

*Do you not know that your body is a temple of the Holy Spirit within you, whom you have from God? You are not your own, for you were bought with a price. So glorify God in your body.*

### 1 Corinthians 6:19-20 (ESV)

Dearest one, I am thrilled to start this next chapter with you. Have you been practicing your new RESOURCE™ tools as we continue to make our way through the acronym RESOURCE™? After this chapter, we move beyond "R" to the rest of our RECON-STRUCTION™ acronym, but for now, we are resourcing our life with tools that stabilize!

Remember, we are mastering RESOURCE™ to ensure we have the skills needed to move into the deeper, more concentrated healing of our inner heart rooms with Jesus. Through RESOURCE™, God is equipping you for the more strenuous parts of your *Heart Journey*™.

Make sure you practice all of your RESOURCE™ tools daily, with special emphasis on those that work well for keeping you in your Window of Tolerance.

To effectively heal and address unmet needs and past traumas, it is vital to cultivate stability in various aspects of our lives, including our mind, emotions, nervous system, and relationships. By expanding our experience of stability, we can create a solid foundation for comfortable and effective healing. Therefore, it is principal to prioritize activities and practices that promote stability, allowing us to engage with healing tools with greater ease and effectiveness.

All of our tools come from the Lord Who is the Healer, and Who is outside of time and able to heal us, restoring what the enemy has taken away in the past, giving us double for our trouble (Isaiah 61:7). Remember the story of Joseph in Genesis? His brothers sold him into slavery, and years later, his family and an entire nation were saved from starvation because of the way God worked in Joseph's life. Like with Joseph, He turns our dysfunctional family woes and painful traumas into fulfilling restoration and His glorious purpose. God is working in you powerfully, but you must also cooperate with Him in the process (Philippians 2:13-14). Keep pressing on. So much good is ahead, Beloved!

Now, with a heart hungry for more of Jesus and His bountiful restoration, we will move ahead with more RESOURCE™ tools. The "O" in RESOURCE™ stands for "Occupy the Body." While on Earth, Jesus inhabited a body, and so do we. I do not believe Jesus walked around with His mind so immersed in the heavens that He forgot He had a body. What is the status of your relationship with your body? Do you love your body the way Jesus does? Do you listen to your body when it speaks to you about its fatigue, needs, and sensations? Can you imagine the Lord, while on Earth, hating or dissociating from His body? I cannot. I believe that while never indulging in the sinful nature, Jesus handled His body with wisdom, love, and faith. He is our model. Take a moment to reflect on your relationship with your body.

Did you know that every emotion you experience is felt in your body? This is because emotions are a neurobiological process that takes place internally within us. They are triggered by our thoughts and perceptions of both internal and external experiences, and they originate in the limbic system, a complex network of interconnected brain structures. The hypothalamus, hippocampus, amygdala, and limbic cortex are all essential components of the brain that contribute to our emotional experiences and resulting behavioral responses. Our sympathetic and parasympathetic nervous systems are highly intertwined with emotions and emotional expression. So, our thoughts can be part of emotional causation, but we perceive our emotions in our soma, our bodies, as sensations. For instance, when we are sad, we often feel "heavy" in our bodies, fear can be felt as "cold feet," and joy can be experienced as a "warm heart."

Interoception, our ability to perceive our internal bodily states and sensations, plays a crucial role in our overall wellness.[9] In order to cultivate this essential skill, we will be learning three specific techniques: grounding, body soothing, and tracking. Through these Occupy the Body skills, we can discover a sense of settled, anchored calm within ourselves and attune to our physical sensations with curiosity and attention. By developing our interoceptive awareness, we can better manage stress and build resilience in the face of challenges.

Below is a brief description of grounding, body soothing, and tracking, and we will be learning to apply these principles through activities in this chapter.[10]

- Grounding: Discovering a settled, anchored, grounded area in the body and, with curiosity, turning your attention to that place. We simultaneously maintain connection with the Lord and His love to our body and experience at the same time.

- Body Soothing: Engaging with real or imagined positive stimuli using one or more of the five senses (e.g., a rose, warm bath water, the scent of cinnamon), and then using curiosity and attention to follow positive sensations in the body after exposure to the stimuli. We simultaneously maintain connection with the Lord and His love to our body and experience at the same time.

- Tracking: Listening with curious attention to the area of the body that is over-activated or under-activated during duress, and following the sensations with curious attention. We simultaneously maintain connection with the Lord and His love to our body and experience at the same time.

In this initial phase of the healing process, grounding, body soothing, and tracking are indispensable skills that provide us with a sense of security and stability within our bodies. As we progress into the memory reconsolidation phase, these skills will be even more crucial in helping us renovate and heal the dilapidated heart rooms in our RECONSTRUCTION™ project.

When we tune in to our bodies, we discover they have their own language, and they communicate just as much as our thoughts. Our bodies can even hold implicit memories, causing them to respond to triggers that our minds may not recognize as potential threats. Through tracking and experiencing our bodily sensations, we can connect with primal levels of awareness, which can be deeply healing.

To move toward healing, it is crucial to become more aware of our bodily sensations while practicing the presence of the Lord at the same time.[11] However, for individuals who have experienced trauma like sexual or physical abuse or severe neglect, connecting with their bodily sensations may prove challenging. Therefore, when engaging in exercises that involve inhabiting the body, it is recommended to find a safe place in the body to which to turn your attention, even if it is a neutral body part like the nose, with fewer nerve endings. It is important to be gentle with yourself and take things at your own pace. And always remember that Jesus, who is safety, is abiding in your body with you (John 15:4). You are never alone, and His love lavishly encases and fills you (Romans 8:31-39).

> *Do you not know that your body is the temple (the very sanctuary) of the Holy Spirit Who lives within you, Whom you have received [as a Gift] from God? You are not your own, You were bought with a price purchased with a preciousness and paid for, made His own. So then, honor God and bring glory to Him in your body.*

### 1 Corinthians 6:19-20 (AMPC)

## TIME TO OCCUPY THE BODY!

Beloved, let us begin our journey of grounding, body soothing, and tracking by taking some time to review a non-exhaustive list of common body sensations. Remember that our emotions are often felt in our bodies, so you may already be experiencing some of these sensations throughout your day. However, the skill of intercepting and identifying these sensations is something you can develop through practice.

Take a moment to tune into your body and see if you can identify any of the sensations on the list. Remember, this is not an all-encompassing list, and everyone may experience sensations differently. Without judgment, simply observe and notice the sensations that arise in your body. This practice will help you become more aware of your bodily responses and emotions, and better equipped to manage them.

| | | | |
|---|---|---|---|
| Achy | Cramped | Heavy | Quivering |
| Airy | Dense | Hot | Radiating |
| Alive | Dizzy | Intense | Ragged |
| Bloated | Dull | Itchy | Raw |
| Blocked | Elastic | Jagged | Rolling |
| Breathless | Electric | Jittery | Shaky |
| Brittle | Empty | Jumbly | Sharp |
| Bubbly | Energized | Knotted | Shimmering |
| Burning | Expanding | Limp | Shivery |
| Buzzing | Flaccid | Lively | Shudder |
| Callous | Fluid | Loose | Silky |
| Chilled | Flushed | Nauseous | Smooth |
| Clammy | Fluttery | Numb | Soft |
| Closed | Frantic | Open | Spacious |
| Cold | Frozen | Paralyzed | Spasming |
| Cuddly | Full | Pounding | Unsteady |
| Constricted | Fuzzy | Prickly | Vibrant |
| Contracted | Goosebumps | Puffy | Warmth |
| Cool | Gurgling | Pulsing | Wrenching |
| Cozy | Harmony | Quaking | Yearning |

Next, we will learn how to use our grounding tool.

## OCCUPY THE BODY: GROUNDING

Grounding is a powerful tool that allows us to connect with positive sensations in our bodies. By using interception to identify and deepen these sensations, we can regulate ourselves and find peace in times of stress. Similarly, anchoring ourselves to these positive sensations can help us stay connected to our bodies and prevent dissociation, which can occur as a result of trauma.

It is important to understand that dissociation from the body is a coping mechanism that can be involuntarily triggered by overwhelming experiences, especially traumatic ones. While it may serve a protective purpose in the moment, it can have negative consequences in the long run, such as increased stress, poor self-care, anxiety, depression, and difficulty connecting with others.

On the other hand, as we become proficient in grounding and anchoring, we can begin to heal and reconnect with our bodies and emotions. In fact, let us try a grounding exercise right now. Go to your *Heart Journey*™ *Journal* and work through the **Grounding Activity.**

Together, we will scan our bodies with curiosity and attention, identifying positive sensations and use them to find stability and peace. This exercise can be a powerful tool in helping you regulate your emotions and feel more present in your body. Time to get started!

Use this QR code to access audible versions of activities.

Well done! I am curious to know if you found that exercise easy, difficult, or somewhere in between. If you found it challenging, please know there are reasons why it may have been difficult. It is common for us to have experienced negative events in our lives that have accustomed us to pain, making it challenging to recognize positive sensations. Additionally, we may hold tension in specific areas of our bodies due to patterns that originated in childhood or past traumas.

That is why it is essential to explore the sensations throughout your entire body, acknowledging and feeling what is there. This practice can help us become more aware of our bodily responses and emotions, and ultimately lead to greater healing and regulation. Hence, keep practicing and remember to be gentle and compassionate with yourself along the way.

Grounding is a vital aspect of our healing journey, and it is normal to struggle with allowing body sensations to move through and out of our bodies. However, by finding an anchor or a place of stability in our bodies, we can become fully present and available to the Lord. This practice can help us downshift our nervous systems, leading to reduced feelings of anxiety, anger, or overwhelm and an increase in positive feelings.

Moreover, reconciling with our bodies and paying attention to our inner life enables us to integrate fully with our bodies and with the Lord. This integration allows us to be used by Him in every aspect of our being, which is both beautiful and powerful. Therefore, let us continue to practice grounding and body awareness, allowing ourselves to become fully present and available to God's love and guidance.

## OCCUPY THE BODY: BODY SOOTHING

Body soothing is very similar to grounding; the only difference is the starting place. With body resourcing, we help ourselves into the process by starting out with a positive stimulus and then move into the body. You can use this tool one of two ways:

1. Body Soothing with Five Senses.

2. Body Soothing with Positive Memory.

Go to your *Heart Journey*™ *Journal* and work through the **Body Soothing Activity.**

Use this QR code to access audible versions of activities.

## OCCUPY THE BODY: TRACKING

Tracking involves lovingly attending to unpleasant body sensations rather than ignoring them. Beloved, it is remarkable to consider that Jesus, as recorded in Luke 22:44 (NKJV), was fully present with His bodily sensations during moments of great emotional distress. The verse reads, "And being in agony, He prayed more earnestly; and His sweat became like great drops of blood falling down to the ground." This shows that even the Son of God experienced bodily responses to His emotions and was fully present with them. In fact, Hebrews 4:15 tells us that Jesus can sympathize with our weaknesses because even He experienced temptation and pain in His body. He was present with His bodily pain, while He was also present with Father God.

As we seek to follow in Jesus' footsteps, we, too, can learn to be fully present with our own emotionally painful bodily sensations during times of distress while practicing the presence of Jesus. The key is developing the capacity to lovingly attend to our body's duress, while fully amalgamating with the presence of the Lord at the same time. In this state of loving attention, full of the heart of God, we track our duress symptoms in our body. Amazingly, under these conditions, negative sensations often shift and move and resolve. While tracking your sensations with the Lord in such a way, it is important to stay out of mental interpretations of your bodily sensations. Instead, just continue to laser focus the love of God on that place and stay in oneness with Jesus.

Remember, tracking and observing our bodily sensations during times of emotional duress can be a powerful tool for managing our nervous system. Negative bodily sensations like a fast heartbeat, tingling in the hands, or nausea are common during stressful situations. By tracking these sensations with curiosity, non-judgment and love, we can learn to make friends with them and manage our nervous system more effectively.

Fear and curiosity cannot coexist, so the more we approach our bodily sensations with a sense of curiosity, the less fear we will feel. As the Scripture says, perfect love casts out all fear (1 John 4:18).

Through the power and love of God, we can listen with loving attention to the areas of our bodies that are over-activated or under-activated during times of emotional duress. By practicing tracking, we can identify the distressing feelings that cause the imbalance and release them. With consistent practice, we can learn to manage our bodily sensations more effectively, leading to greater peace in our lives.

As you practice tracking, remember to remain curious and try to not narrate a story of why you feel what you feel. Just be with the sensations as you are also with Jesus. If at any time it feels like too much, stop and turn your attention to your grounding/anchoring sensations or go do something fun.

Take time now to go to your *Heart Journey™ Journal* and work through the **Tracking Activity.**

Use this QR code to access audible versions of activities.

I am proud of you for taking the time to practice grounding, body soothing, and tracking. Remember, progress is not always linear, and it is essential to celebrate any effort you make toward wholeness. Consistent practice of these skills can assist you in managing your emotions more effectively and finding greater peace in your life. Keep up the good effort, as these skills will be essential to our upcoming work together. Practice grounding, body soothing, and tracking daily!

## OCCUPY THE BODY: TRIGGERS

It is normal to have triggers that can bring up intense emotional or physical reactions, especially when associated with past traumatic experiences. A trigger refers to any stimulus or event that brings up acute emotional or physical reactions, often associated with past traumatic experiences. These triggers can range from a particular smell or sound, to a specific situation or memory. Sometimes, even a simple thought can trigger us into experiencing emotional pain, as if the past trauma is present in the current situation. Triggers can cause us to feel overwhelmed, anxious, or even reexperience past traumatic events.

In the second chapter, we delved into the concept of the Window of Tolerance, which represents our optimal zone for effectively managing triggers and stressors. A healthy nervous system maintains a harmonious equilibrium between the sympathetic and parasympathetic systems, smoothly transitioning between them throughout the day, without veering into extremes such as fight, flight, freeze, or collapse responses. This is our goal.

## OCCUPY THE BODY: AWARENESS OF ORIENTING, STARTLING, AND DEFENSIVE RESPONSES

We can also be aware of our somatic responses, such as orienting, startle, and defensive responses. In the next chapter we will work with these responses as we practice Time Reversing Trauma™.

Orienting responses happen when we become aware of a new stimulus in our environment. For example, if you hear a noise while walking in the woods, your body may turn your head and orient your ears toward the sound to better understand where it came from. In the Bible, we see an example of an orienting response in the story of Moses and the burning bush. When Moses saw the bush on fire, he turned toward it to understand what was happening (Exodus 3:3-4). When we have experienced much trauma, we can demonstrate dull orienting responses (dissociation) or overactive orienting responses (hypervigilance). As we move into more wholeness, so does our orienting response.

Startle responses occur when we are suddenly surprised or scared. For instance, if someone jumps at you from behind a corner, your body may react by quickly jumping back or tightening up. An example of a startle response in the Bible is when King Saul threw a spear at David, and David involuntarily dodged it quickly (1 Samuel 18:10-11). Similar to the orienting response, the startle response can be overactive or dulled as a response to trauma. Trauma recovery will bring the startle response back into normalcy.

Defensive responses are activated when we feel threatened or in danger. These responses are usually more intense and involve a fight, flight, or freeze response. In the Bible, we see examples of defensive responses in the story of David and Goliath, where David fought against Goliath to defend his people (1 Samuel 17:41-51). Triggers can often lead us to respond defensively, but as we work through healing unmet needs and processing trauma in the upcoming chapters, we can bring our defensive responses back into proper balance.

In this section, on Occupy the Body, I introduced somatic nervous system tools and concepts that will be essential in the upcoming chapters. Understanding somatic responses will play a significant role in our work. It is crucial to identify triggers and utilize our RESOURCE™ tools effectively to manage them, promote emotional regulation, and reduce nervous system distress. As we progress through our study, we will encounter Jesus in these triggers, and He will bring restoration. Through the *Heart Journey*™, we can expand our Window of Tolerance by utilizing regulating tools and experiencing healing, thus restoring emotional wholeness.

Now open your *Heart Journey*™ *Journal* and work through the **Individual Heartwork - Occupy the Body.**

## UNDERGIRD WITH SUPPORT.

As we move through our *Heart Journey*™ and move toward rebuilding and transforming the rooms within us, it is imperative to have a solid support system in place. The RESOURCE™ acronym's "U" stands for "Undergird with Support," highlighting the importance of social nourishment. As Christians, we understand that we need each other, as God said, "It's not good that the human is alone," Genesis 2:18 (CEB). Research equally shows the significance of having close relationships with safe people. Healthy relationships regulate our nervous system as relational nutrition to our heart, our deepest core.

## CO-REGULATION

We are made to co-regulate with the Lord and with safe others. Neuropsychological research shows that healthy relationships with safe others provide us with the necessary emotional and physiological support to regulate our nervous system. Co-regulation refers to the process of regulating one's nervous system through the support and influence of another person. It is a reciprocal process where two or more individuals attune to each other's emotional and physiological states, and work together to regulate and stabilize their nervous systems. When we co-regulate with others, our brains release hormones that help us feel calm, safe, and connected, which in turn supports our overall well-being.

The Father formed our brains to prioritize social interactions not only for our survival, but also for our fulfillment and joy. Co-regulating with Him and with safe others is His lavish gift for our minds, bodies, and souls, allowing us to experience the richness of deep and meaningful relationships as a home for our hearts.

Our heart home has been grooved and fashioned by our childhood experiences, whether positive or negative. When we faced trauma and unmet needs in our younger years, we often felt alone and isolated. Take our friend, Deborah, for instance. Even when surrounded by family members on special occasions, the adults usually did not engage with her emotionally. As a result, she rarely felt they heard her or even cared about her. To Deborah, their interactions with her seemed to focus on what they could get out of her, not how they could love and support her emotionally. Furthermore, in the aftermath of recurring episodes of violence within the family home, she experienced an amplified sense of isolation and profound loneliness in her anguish, longing for someone to embrace the depths of her heartache.

For some of us, even though we had caring adults present during challenging times, we still experienced a deep-seated loneliness, yearning for someone who could truly listen, accept, validate, and offer solace, but perhaps due to their own limitations or lack of relational skills, they were unable to meet those needs. For instance, Katy's story helps us understand how a lack of validation, understanding and co-regulation in childhood can happen innocently. During Katy's childhood, her mother's prolonged illness placed a significant burden on her father, leaving him unable to fully address Katy's emotional needs. Additionally, Katy's mother's own health challenges prevented her from providing the emotional support Katy longed for. Despite growing up in a loving Christian family, Katy now grapples with a profound sense of loneliness in her adult life.

Irrespective of the experiences you had during your childhood, it is necessary to develop the ability to skillfully connect with safe individuals in your present reality. Building relationships with trustworthy and supportive people is not only essential for your overall well-being, but it becomes even more significant as you embark on the journey of healing from these challenging experiences. Surrounding yourself with a loving and wholehearted social support system creates a container through which God's love can flow, as these individuals stand by you and hold you during your healing process.

*I led them with cords of human kindness, with ties of love.*
*To them I was like one who lifts a little child to the cheek,*
*and I bent down to feed them.*

Hosea 11:4 (NIV)

## UNDERGIRD WITH SUPPORT: IDENTIFY SAFE PEOPLE

The first rung to crossing over into meaningful connection with safe people is defining safety. Who should we consider as a safe person? While the safest person is undoubtedly our glorious Lord Himself, safe individuals exhibit qualities such as kindness, consistency, forgiveness, and effective communication skills. They are also self-aware and willing to acknowledge their mistakes and offer sincere apologies when needed. Before you identify who is safe in your life, be sure to take inventory of your own person. Safe people attract safe people, so the "safer" you become, the easier it will be to draw safe relationships into your life.

It is essential to understand that safe people can still experience conflicts, just like everyone else. Conflict has been present since the first family, after all. However, safe people possess the emotional capacity to navigate these conflicts in a healthy way. They work through issues and are able to forgive and proceed forward. Safe individuals do not cause harm or instill fear, and they are supportive when we need them. That is why, it is essential to surround ourselves with safe and available individuals whenever possible.

Here are fourteen characteristics of safe others:

1. Honesty: Safe people are truthful and honest with themselves and others.

2. Empathy: Safe people are empathetic and can put themselves in other people's shoes. They are sensitive to others' feelings and experiences.

3. Dependability: Safe people are reliable and dependable. They keep their promises and follow through on commitments.

4. Boundaries: Safe people know and respect their own boundaries, as well as others' boundaries. They do not overstep or manipulate.

5. Accountability: Safe people take responsibility for their actions and behaviors. They own their mistakes and apologize when necessary.

6. Non-judgmental: Safe people are non-judgmental and accepting. They do not shame or criticize others for their thoughts, feelings, or actions.

7. Supportive: Safe people are supportive and encouraging. They provide emotional support and are willing to help.

8. Confidentiality: Safe people keep confidences and do not gossip or share personal information without permission.

9. Respectful: Safe people are respectful and considerate of others' feelings and opinions. They do not dismiss or invalidate others.

10. Kindness: Safe people are kind and compassionate toward others, showing empathy and understanding.

11. Consistency: Safe people are consistent in their behaviors and actions, providing a sense of stability and predictability.

12. Self-awareness: Safe people are self-aware, recognizing their own strengths and weaknesses and how they impact others.

13. Good communication skills: Safe people demonstrate good communication skills, allowing for clear and effective communication.

14. Forgiving: Safe people are forgiving and do not hold grudges. They are willing to work through conflicts and move forward.

Safe people provide a secure and supportive environment where we feel seen, heard, and validated. Jesus exemplifies these qualities and offers us unconditional love and grace. In the presence of safe people, we experience a glimpse of Jesus' love and compassion.

## AVAILABILITY

To establish an effective connection, both parties need to be available. For a connection to be truly powerful, both parties must be willing to make sacrifices and prioritize the relationship. It is worth noting that just because someone seems safe, it does not mean they have the time or emotional capacity to provide full or reciprocal support. In such cases, we should graciously look for a few individuals who can be there for us when we need them most, instead of relying on just one person.

It is important to remember that even people we trust might not be able to provide the emotional support we crave during difficult times. In these situations, joining support groups like Cleansing Streams, Grief Share, Divorce Care, Celebrate Recovery, Al-Anon meetings, Bible Studies, or other recovery meetings can help us expand our support network and receive the emotional support we need. If we cannot find these groups in our local church, we might need to look elsewhere, such as online communities.

If you are taking this *Heart Journey*™ with a small group, lean on your fellow sisters in Christ for support. If you are not on this journey with fellow Christians, consider seeking a licensed psychotherapist who is experienced in treating trauma and who shares your worldview or is Christian-friendly. A competent psychotherapist will respect your worldview and collaborate with you based on your values and goals. Make sure to communicate your values and worldview to any mental health professional providing you with treatment.

Additionally, it is essential to draw closer to the Lord during this time. He wants to support, sustain, and champion you, deeply and profoundly. God is your primary attachment figure, and we can rely on Him for provision. He has created us in His image and has both paternal and maternal characteristics, making Him a wonderful parent Who is loving and nurturing in every way possible. Nevertheless, if you have experienced trauma that has impacted your sense of safety with the Lord, start with small steps like reading Scriptures that speak of God's love and goodness to facilitate your connection with Him.

## UNDERGIRD WITH SUPPORT: SOCIALGRAM™

You are about to work on your Socialgram™ and identify your current support structure. Then you will work toward increasing safe support in your life. To ensure you have adequate support, aim to cultivate relationships with at least six safe individuals in your two inner Socialgram™ circles, i.e., those who are closest to you and available to spend time with you. A good recommendation is to check in with several of these safe others weekly.

It is time to go to your *Heart Journey*™ *Journal*. First you will determine how safe of a person you are. Then you will create a Socialgram™, which will help you map out your social support network. Go to **Individual Heartwork - Undergird with Support.**

## RELAXATION SKILLS

Relaxation skills work directly with our physiology and help us calm our nervous system. The RESOURCE™ acronym's "R" stands for "Relax the Body," which is especially important within today's fast-paced world. As women, we often wearily carry the weight of multiple responsibilities on our shoulders, which can make it challenging to take time for ourselves and truly disentangle and unwind. However, relaxation is key to "resourcing" ourselves from a cognitive, spiritual, and physiological perspective.

In these exercises, we will focus on the physiological aspect of relaxation and how to calm our bodies when we feel overwhelmed. Women experience unique physical and emotional stressors that can affect their bodies differently than men. For instance, for many of us, hormonal fluctuations throughout the menstrual cycle and life stages like pregnancy and menopause can influence our response to stress and impact our physical and emotional well-being in distinct ways. Moreover, societal pressures often place a heavier burden on women, particularly in terms of caretaking responsibilities, which further contributes to their unique experience of stress. Additionally, we tend to hold trauma in our bodies as physical duress. Relaxation techniques can directly address this bodily duress.

We will use various tools to achieve physiological relaxation, such as progressive muscle relaxation, deep breathing, sensory grounding techniques, and a meditation called "5, 4, 3, 2, 1." As we learn these skills, we will be keenly focused on the breath of God.

In the Bible, one of the Hebrew words for breath is "Ruach," which can also mean wind or spirit, representing God's active presence in our lives. In Ezekiel 37:9-10 (NKJV), the prophet Ezekiel has a vision of the valley of dry bones, symbolizing a spiritually dead and lifeless condition. In this vision, God instructs Ezekiel to prophesy to the bones, saying, "Thus says the Lord God: 'Come from the four winds, O breath (Ruach), and breathe on these slain, that they may live.'" As Ezekiel prophesies, the breath of God (Ruach) enters the bones, causing them to come to life, with flesh and skin covering them. This vivid depiction illustrates the power of God's Spirit (Ruach) to bring about transformation, restoration, and new life even in the most hopeless, dry, and death-filled situations.

Additionally, the word "Neshemah" is used to describe the breath of life God breathed into Adam, giving him life. We find this in Genesis 2:7 (NKJV), which states, "And the Lord God formed man of the dust of the ground, and breathed into his nostrils the breath of life; and man became a living being." Here, "Neshemah Chayim" represents the life-giving breath of God, emphasizing His role as the source of life for humanity. These words remind us the breath of God is essential to our existence and has the power to calm, sustain, fill, and empower us.

Moreover, in Psalm 46:10 (NIV), we are instructed to "be still and know that I am God." This stillness involves taking deep breaths and focusing on the presence of God within us. In John 20:22 (NIV), Jesus breathes on His disciples and says, "Receive the Holy Spirit." This breath from Jesus fills His followers with the power and Presence of the Holy Spirit.

As we practice relaxation techniques, we will breathe in the breath of God, allowing Him to calm, sustain, fill, and empower us. Our first tool is "Christian Progressive Relaxation."

## RELAXATION SKILLS: CHRISTIAN PROGRESSIVE RELAXATION

Progressive muscle relaxation is a technique that reverses the body's physiological response to stress, by intentionally tensing and releasing specific muscle groups. By tensing the muscles beyond their current state of constriction due to duress, we create space for the muscles to release and de-stress even further, resulting in a deep sense of relaxation in the body. This process decreases muscle tension, slows heart rate, and reduces blood pressure, leading to a calmer state of mind and body. It also decreases the levels of stress hormones such as cortisol and adrenaline, resulting in a more relaxed and tranquil bodily state. It is essential to listen to your body during this exercise and stop immediately if you experience any pain or discomfort. Allow the Holy Spirit to guide you through this process of relaxation and healing.

Take time now to go to your *Heart Journey*™ *Journal* and work through the **Christian Progressive Relaxation Activity.**

Use this QR code to access audible versions of activities.

## RELAXATION SKILLS: CHRISTIAN DIAPHRAGMATIC BREATHING

Next, we will learn "Diaphragmatic Breathing" which is also known as belly breathing or deep breathing. This type of breathing can help you feel more relaxed, reduce stress and anxiety, and even lower your heart rate and blood pressure. Again, we will breathe in the Ruach of God using our holy imagination.

Take time now to go to your *Heart Journey*™ *Journal* and work through the **Christian Diaphragmatic Breathing Activity.**

Use this QR code to access audible versions of activities.

## RELAXATION SKILLS: CHRISTIAN FOUR SQUARE BREATHING

Another effective technique for managing anxiety is called "Four Square Breathing." It involves taking a deep breath in through your nose for four counts, then holding that breath for four counts. Next, slowly exhale for four counts, and then hold your breath out for another four counts. While doing this, you can visualize drawing a square in your mind or on paper to help focus your attention. It is important to practice this technique regularly, even when you are not feeling anxious, so your mind and body become familiar with it. This way, when you do experience anxiety, you will be able to use the technique with ease and confidence.

Take time now to go to your *Heart Journey*™ *Journal* and work through the **Christian Four Square Breathing Activity.**

Use this QR code to access audible versions of activities.

## RELAXATION SKILLS: CHRISTIAN BODY SCAN

Our next relaxation tool is "Christian Body Scan." In this activity, tune in to your body and invite the Holy Spirit to guide you. Start by finding a comfortable seated position with your feet planted firmly on the ground.

Take time now to go to your *Heart Journey*™ *Journal* and work through the **Christian Body Scan Activity.**

Use this QR code to access audible versions of activities.

## RELAXATION SKILLS: 5, 4, 3, 2, 1 MEDITATION-CHRISTIAN VERSION

The "5, 4, 3, 2, 1 Meditation Christian Version" is a popular contemplative activity that again uses your holy imagination and focuses on your five senses and gratitude. Our senses are always in the present moment, and when we feel fearful, it is because our mind is focused on the future or the past. This activity will help us focus on the present and also on the Lord (Matthew 6:34).

Now go to your *Heart Journey™ Journal* and start the meditation called **5, 4, 3, 2, 1 Meditation-Christian Version Activity.**

Use this QR code to access audible versions of activities.

## COMFORT THROUGH SELF-MOMMING™!

As we continue to RESOURCE™ ourselves, we will look at the letter "C" for "Comfort through Self-Momming™." Self-Momming™ gives us a way to meet our needs that were not met in childhood now, in the current day. We will use Jesus as our model parent.

As we examine the Scripture, we see how Jesus lovingly parents us deep in our inner heart, almost like a nurturing maternal figure.[12] In Psalm 139, we are reminded that we are fearfully and wonderfully made and that God knit us together in our mother's womb. Jesus, our Good Shepherd, knows us intimately and cares for us deeply and with profound nurturing. Like a mother, He seeks to save every lost place in our heart homes. He desires to nurture and guide us, providing comfort and encouragement during times of struggle. In Isaiah 66:13, we are told that God comforts us as a mother comforts her child, and in Matthew 23:37, Jesus speaks of gathering His people like a mother hen gathers her chicks under her wings. Through these passages, we can see how Jesus tenderly parents us, providing a sense of safety and security in His love. We can trust that Jesus is always with us, nurturing us in the deepest places of our hearts (Luke 19:10; Revelation 3:20).

The Self-Momming™ tool will help us achieve more oneness with Jesus at our center. We will take His hand and learn to be one with Him, using our holy imagination to nurture ourselves as a loving mother in oneness with Him. But why do we need Self-Momming™?

As adult women, we ultimately become our own parent, right? We are the ones who have to tell ourselves, "No, you are not going to eat out because there is food at home," and "You need to brush your teeth before bed." Or we might need to say, "You have not budgeted money for that," or "This dessert is not healthy for your body." So as adults, we find that we have to lead ourselves like a parent would a child. Unfortunately, most of us have internalized an extremely punitive inner critic rather than a nurturing and wise parent.

The rejection we all experience in the world, the enemy's insistent twisting lies from the unseen realm, and the shame inherent in humanity from the garden can culminate together to form an internal oppressive and deafening dictator that is difficult to tolerate. Our inner world is like a garden, and without constant care, it will quickly become overgrown with the weeds of ungodly self-criticism. We need to skillfully replace this tyrannical voice with an internal, wise and nurturing parent that is governed by the love and wisdom of God.

Over time, we have developed enough nurturing skills to cultivate many relationships with friends, family, church members, other professionals, clients, pets, mentees, and perhaps our own children. Beloved, now it is time to nurture ourselves! But how do we do that?

Here is how. When you encounter a stressful situation, take a moment to ask Jesus what He has to say to you about the situation. Ask, "Jesus, how do You want to parent me in this situation?" Then, let Him speak to you as you take His hand. Be aware of His voice coming to you in a new way. As you listen to Him, check all around the periphery of your spiritual awareness to ensure openness to hearing Him. Remember, His sheep hear His voice. Then, nourish your inner child by speaking from your most adult self with His love as your source and example. Become one with Him as you listen to, understand, and accept your inner vulnerable self. Speak words of life to the parts of you that feel shame, defeat, or rejection. Imagine what an ideal mother would say to you, and allow yourself to feel comfort, validation, love, and acceptance, drawing strength from Jesus' power and example.

It is not enough to simply receive nurturing from Him; you must also participate and agree with His nurturing by treating yourself the same way. HEARing stands for "hearing, empathizing, accepting, and respecting." Just like you must demonstrate HEARing your significant other, you must also demonstrate HEARing all the parts of you, and especially your vulnerable parts of self.

## SELF-MOMMING™ ACTIVITY

Deborah experienced amazing breakthroughs as she practiced Self-Momming™. She had been struggling with a harsh inner critic, which mirrored the criticism she grew up with, and had internalized rejection and negative thoughts. Upon discovering the Self-Momming™ tool, Deborah used the nurturing example of her childhood neighbor's mother, Mrs. Swallow, as a model for how to treat herself with kindness and compassion. She also drew inspiration from the tenderness she often felt from Jesus during her morning devotions. By making time for Self-Momming™ daily and using these models, Deborah was able to nurture her inner child and experienced a positive change in her mood and confidence.

In summary, Self-Momming™ is a tool that enables us to meet the needs that were not met in childhood by nurturing ourselves in oneness with Jesus. It helps us replace the harsh inner critic with a nurturing and wise parent who is governed by the love and wisdom of God. By asking Jesus how He wants to parent us in a situation and listening to His nurturing and wise words, we can comfort and encourage ourselves during times of struggle. We can then speak the words of life to ourselves, drawing strength from Jesus' power and example. Self-Momming™ is a skill that requires participation and agreement with Jesus' nurturing, just like demonstrating love to a significant other. By practicing Self-Momming™, we can cultivate emotional safety and allow Jesus to parent us deeply in the inner chambers of our hearts.

Take time now to go to your *Heart Journey™ Journal* and work through the **Individual Heartwork - Comfort Through the Self-Momming™ Activity** and **Individual Heartwork Relaxation** and **Self - Momming™ Reflection.**

Use this QR code to access audible versions of activities.

## ENLIGHTEN WITH CONTENT

The last piece of our RESOURCE™ acronym is "E" for "Enlighten with Content." It is fascinating how what we listen to can greatly impact our mind, emotions, and ultimately, the direction of our lives. Science has shown that listening to positive and uplifting content can lead to an increase in feelings of happiness, motivation, and resilience.[13] On the other hand, constantly exposing ourselves to negative and destructive content can have detrimental effects on our mental, emotional, and relational well-being.

Again, in Philippians 4:8, Paul encourages us to focus on things that are true, noble, right, pure, lovely, admirable, excellent, and praiseworthy. When we intentionally seek out positive and healing content, we align ourselves with this biblical principle. We choose to fill our minds with things that uplift and edify, rather than allow negativity and despair to take root.

On our *Heart Journey*™ toward healing, it is imperative that we actively seek out resources that aid us in our process. We must be diligent in finding podcasts, talks, audiobooks, and videos that speak to our hearts and inspire us to keep moving forward. Let positive content create a healing cocoon around your mind, and allow the Holy Spirit to transform your thinking and emotions.

It is important to note that as we spend more time reading, listening to, and meditating on the Word of God, our minds can enter into a state of peace and wisdom. The Bible tells us in Psalm 119:105 that God's Word is a lamp to our feet and a light to our path. When we meditate on the Word, we allow its truths to permeate our minds, renewing our thoughts, and transforming our hearts. This leads to a deeper understanding of God's will and purpose for our lives, as well as a greater sense of peace and joy in all circumstances. As we focus on God's promises and His character, our perspective shifts from one of fear and anxiety, to one of trust and confidence in His faithfulness. So let us make it a priority to regularly immerse ourselves in God's Word, allowing it to guide our thoughts and shape our lives.

Furthermore, as we continue to surround ourselves with recovery content and support, we must be discerning in what we engage with. It is important the content aligns with our values and beliefs in the Lord. In Proverbs 4:23, we are reminded to guard our hearts above all else, for everything we do flows from it. Let us intentionally choose to fill our minds and hearts with positive and uplifting content, allowing it to shape the course of our lives toward healing and wholeness.

In addition to filling our minds with positive content, it is essential to understand how our nervous system responds to what we listen to. Our nervous system is responsible for regulating our body's response to stress and trauma. When we listen to negative and destructive content, our nervous system can become dysregulated, leading to symptoms such as anxiety, depression, and even physical ailments. However, when we intentionally seek out positive and uplifting content, our nervous system regulates, leading to feelings of calm, safety, and relaxation.

As we continue on our *Heart Journey*™ toward healing, let us be mindful of what we expose ourselves to, knowing it can have a significant impact on our overall well-being.

Take time now to go to your *Heart Journey*™ *Journal* and work through the **Heartwork for Enlighten with Content.**

## EDIT OUT NEGATIVE CONTENT

Likewise, just as it is important to increase the level of positive content with which you are filling your heart and mind, it is equally important to edit out negative content. We will be working on healing your attachment system, decreasing fear, and reducing distress. Therefore, it is vital you edit out the voices and entertainment that put you in a state of distress. For example, if you have a goal to reduce fear, it is essential you avoid watching anxiety-provoking streaming content.

Take time now to go to your *Heart Journey*™ *Journal* and complete the **Individual Heartwork - Restoring My Nervous System** and **Heart Group Discussion - Time to Share.**

## YOUR GROWING TOOL BELT

Beloved, I am proud of your faithfulness and the progress you have made in gaining tools for your *Heart Journey*™. After completing the Heartwork for this chapter, we will focus on addressing our behavioral habits that hinder our healing, and then surge into heart reconstruction tools that will deeply impact your life. Here is the list of *Heart Journey*™ stabilization tools you have practiced so far.

1. Reframe by Inventorying Your Thinking

2. Reframe through Mind Mansion™

3. Reframe through Daily Journal Practice

4. Enrich with Positive Memories

5. Uncoupling Exercise

6. Enrich with Safe Place Imagery

7. Enrich with Eyes of Jesus™

8. Structure Your Life: Self-care

9. Structure Your Life: Life Edit

10. Structure Your Life: Seven Types of Rest

11. Occupy the Body: Grounding

12. Occupy the Body: Body Soothing

13. Occupy the Body: Tracking

14. Undergird with Support: Identify Safe People

15. Undergird with Support: Socialgram™

16. Relaxation Skills: Christian Progressive Relaxation

17. Relaxation Skills: Christian Diaphragmatic Breathing

18. Relaxation Skills: Christian Four Square Breathing

19. Relaxation Skills: Christian Body Scan

20. Relaxation Skills: 5, 4, 3, 2, 1 Meditation-Christian Version

21. Comfort through Self-Momming™!

22. Enlighten with Content

Wow! You have come so far already! I am praying for you right now as I write this, and more importantly, know, Beloved, Jesus is with you every step of the way. Keep pushing forward, because there are so many great things that are waiting for you on the other side. And practice your tools daily!

## LET US PRAY.

*Heavenly Father,*

*Thank You that we can begin healing our hearts and be renewed in Christ. Father, we love the idea of being used by You more and more every day, but we know, in order to do so, our hearts must be turned toward You, and we must be willing for You to do your work in us. Lord, make our hearts malleable. And if there is a shambled area of our hearts where we do not see a need for renovation, Father, please guide us in Your gentle way toward complete restoration.*

*In Jesus' name, Amen.*

# *Chapter*

## FOUR
### Restoring My Healthy Habits

*But the fruit of the Spirit is love, joy, peace, patience, kindness, goodness, faithfulness, gentleness, self-control; against such things there is no law.*
### Galatians 5:22-23 (ESV)

In continuing our *Heart Journey*™, we are preparing the property of our hearts for the RECONSTRUCTION™ process. We just wrapped up the "R" for the acronym RECONSTRUCTION™. The "R" helped us learn to "RESOURCE™," another acronym. Now we move on to the "E" in RECONSTRUCTION™, which stands for "Eliminate Unhelpful Behaviors." Together we will remove the behavioral stumbling blocks in the way of our healing.

## UNHELPFUL BEHAVIORS

Each of us has our own unhelpful behaviors that may stem from past trauma. During our childhood, we may have developed certain patterns of behavior that helped us cope with challenging emotions like anxiety, depression, post-traumatic stress, and flashbacks, which led to issues like substance abuse, addiction, control, disordered eating, and the like.

This is the stage in our journey where we focus on curbing those unhelpful behaviors, substituting them with more beneficial ones. The goal is to allow ourselves to feel emotions genuinely, without resorting to artificial means, escape, or control that have consumed too much of our time and energy. Essentially, we aim to replace these behaviors with healthy coping mechanisms, so we can move on to doing deeper Heartwork.

Let me give you an example. Drinking alcohol is not inherently bad if used in moderation. However, when we use it to numb our feelings or get drunk, it can become harmful. While substances like alcohol can help us relax, we need to be mindful of addictive patterns that can develop. But at the same time, we all need to experience relaxation, comfort, and peace, especially after a stressful day.

An occasional drink of alcohol in moderation is not necessarily detrimental to our well-being. Similarly, an occasional cinnamon bun is harmless. However, excessive consumption of alcohol, cinnamon buns, or other substances to escape from emotions can become problematic. While substances like alcohol may initially provide a sense of relaxation and comfort, developing addictive tendencies can ultimately do more harm than good. Nonetheless, the desire for relaxation and comfort remains valid and needs to be addressed in healthy ways. This is where replacement behaviors are beneficial. We learn to find healthy alternatives that give us the same positive effects without the negative consequences.

In order to lead a healthier, happier, and God-centered life, it is important to take a moment to reflect on any unhealthy coping mechanisms we may be using. While pleasure center activities like eating sweets, social media scrolling, and shopping can be enjoyable and beneficial when used in moderation, it is important to understand the impact they can have on our brain when used excessively.

The pleasure center in our brain is a complex network of structures, with the nucleus accumbens being the main player. When we engage in pleasurable activities, dopamine is released in this area, which gives us a sense of pleasure and reinforces the behavior. However, when we use these behaviors as a way to cope with difficult emotions or stress, it can become problematic and lead to addiction and excess.

For example, gambling can activate the pleasure center and lead to addiction, as people become dependent on the rush of winning. Hoarding can also activate the pleasure center, as people feel a sense of reward or satisfaction from collecting items, even if they are not necessary. Similarly, sleeping too much or spending too much time in bed can be a way of avoiding difficult emotions or responsibilities.

If we notice that we are engaging in any of these behaviors to an excessive or out of control degree, it is important to examine them and understand why they are happening. By identifying the underlying causes and finding healthier ways to cope, we can replace these behaviors and lead a more fulfilling life.

Additionally, when we rely on addictive behaviors to escape or avoid difficult emotions or situations, it becomes challenging to address the root causes of our issues. This can lead to being stuck in a cycle of using addictive behaviors to cope instead of addressing the underlying problems. Therefore, it is important to recognize these patterns, and work on replacing them with healthier coping mechanisms to move forward in our personal growth and healing journey.

## DEBORAH'S STORY

Deborah's story is a great example of how coping mechanisms can manifest from unmet needs and traumas, and that identifying and addressing them can lead to positive changes. Deborah struggled with her mother's alcoholism and the absence of her father, and found comfort in food. However, she soon realized that her excessive eating and poor food choices were actually part of a harmful cycle of food obsession, compulsive eating, and shame.

Through her *Heart Journey*™ work and with the support of her accountability partners and faith, Deborah was able to break this cycle and adopt healthier habits. She made better food choices that nourished her body and used replacement behaviors, such as calling a prayer partner and praying together, when tempted. As a result, she started feeling healthier, more energetic, and emotionally stable.

Deborah's positive changes in her food habits not only contributed to her overall emotional well-being, but also helped her achieve professional success and happiness. She also experienced more intimacy with the Lord as she turned to Him rather than to food for comfort when triggered. Most importantly, she was no longer using food to escape from her difficult emotions. Deborah's story shows that with determination, support, and the right tools, we can break harmful coping mechanisms and lead happier and healthier lives.

Beloved, when we examine our unhealthy behaviors, it is important to understand that they did not just appear out of nowhere. There is a reason why we started engaging in a self-sabotaging behavior, even though it ultimately hurts us. It served a purpose at one point in our lives, whether it was to escape from difficult emotions or gain a sense of control. The problem is that this behavior is no longer serving us and can lead to various problems.

So, what can we do about it? One approach is to conduct a "Behavioral Chain Analysis" or "BCA," which is a helpful tool to examine our behavior and identify the underlying triggers and consequences. Dear one, this activity will guide you through the process of conducting a BCA to gain a better understanding of your behavior and its impact on your life. God is standing by to deliver us.

> *Wretched and miserable man that I am! Who will [rescue me and] set me free from this body of death [this corrupt, mortal existence]? Thanks be to God [for my deliverance] through Jesus Christ our Lord! So then, on the one hand I myself with my mind serve the law of God, but on the other, with my flesh [my human nature, my worldliness, my sinful capacity—I serve] the law of sin.*
>
> **Romans 7:24-25 (AMP)**

## BEHAVIORAL CHAIN ANALYSIS (BCA)

A Behavior Chain Analysis (BCA) can help us understand the different elements that contribute to a behavior and enable us to make more helpful choices in the future. To start with, we should take some time to pray and reflect on what behavior is holding us back from healing. Which behaviors are we using as a coping mechanism to escape or control, and what is it that prevents us from facing our true emotions?

We will use an insightful tool called Behavior Chain Analysis (BCA) to gain a deeper understanding of our self-sabotaging behaviors. BCA involves breaking down a behavior into smaller components, such as setting events, triggers, thoughts, and consequences, to identify the root causes of the behavior. By doing so, we can discover patterns and connections that may not have been immediately apparent, and develop new strategies to overcome them.

After we identify the troublesome behavior we desire to address, we can start looking for "setting events" that might make it more likely to happen. Setting events refer to the conditions or factors that increase the likelihood of a specific behavior occurring. These events are not the cause of the behavior, but rather contribute to the occurrence of the behavior. Setting events may include physical or emotional factors such as lack of sleep, stress, hunger, or feeling overwhelmed. For example, imagine someone is trying to quit smoking, but they find themselves smoking when they experience stress at work. In this case, the stressful situation could be considered a setting event that increases the likelihood of the person smoking. By identifying and addressing the setting event, such as developing healthy coping mechanisms for dealing with work stress, the person may be able to reduce their urge to smoke and successfully quit.

Setting events can be related to our health, hormones, or any other factors that may have set us up to indulge in the behavior. We need to understand that the behavior is not the fault of the setting event, but rather, it may have made us more susceptible to self-sabotaging behaviors.

We will also explore and write down what happened immediately preceding the problematic behavior. This allows us to identify the specific trigger that set off the behavior. We then explore each step of the chain of events that led up to the final consequences of the behavior. This includes examining the thoughts and emotions that arose during each step and how they contributed to the behavior.

In addition to identifying setting events and triggers, it is important to understand the functions of our behaviors. There are four primary functions of behavior, commonly known as S.E.A.T: sensory, escape, attention, and tangible.

Behaviors with a sensory function are those that provide sensory stimulation or pleasure, such as the taste of goodies while overeating or the sensation experienced while over-using alcohol. Behaviors with the function of escape are used to avoid uncomfortable situations or emotions, such as withdrawing from social situations or using drugs to numb feelings. Attention-seeking behaviors are used to gain attention or recognition from others whether positive or negative, such as acting out or creating drama. Behaviors with the function of gaining access to tangibles involve obtaining tangible objects, such as over-shopping, stealing, or hoarding.

Once we have identified the function of the behavior, we can work on finding a replacement behavior that serves the same function but in a more positive, healthy and God-honoring way. For example, if someone engages in overeating as a sensory seeking behavior, they may be able to find a replacement behavior such as chewing gum or lighting a scented candle while in a bubble bath to provide similarly soothing sensory stimulation. If someone uses substances to escape uncomfortable emotions, they may benefit from learning healthy coping mechanisms such as our Christian relaxation tools from Chapter Three.

It is important to keep in mind that finding a replacement behavior that serves the same function is central for success in changing behavior patterns. The replacement behavior needs to be a viable alternative that meets the same needs as the problem behavior. It may take some experimentation and trial and error to find the right replacement behavior, but the effort is worth it in the end.

By analyzing our behaviors in this way, we gain valuable insights into our patterns of thinking and behaving. This can help us to identify any unhealthy coping mechanisms we may be using and find new, more positive ways to deal with difficult emotions. Ultimately, BCA helps us to break free from the cycle of self-sabotage and make positive changes in our lives. Our BCA work will enable us to be better doers of the word (James 1:22-25).

"Let us explore Lydia's story. Suppose Lydia had a stressful day at work, and after her husband went to bed, she decided to drink a bottle of wine." She thought she could finish the open bottle without him noticing. She started with one glass, but then kept going until she finished the whole bottle and even opened another one. The next day, she felt not only hungover, but also guilty, and she confessed to her husband what happened. Although he forgave her, she still struggled to forgive herself and felt distant from God for a few days.

To analyze this situation using a BCA, we start by identifying the setting events and breaking down the chain of events that led to the behavior. We look at the pre-temptation and temptation stages, the behavior itself, and the resolution of the scenario. Here are steps you will take:

1. Identify and write down the setting events.

2. Identify and write down the trigger.

3. Identify and write down each step that occurs after the trigger.

4. Identify and write down how you felt at each point.

5. Review the chain of events and emotions and write down where you could have intervened to change the outcome.

6. Explore and name the functioning behavior.

7. Come up with a replacement behavior.

In Lydia's example, here is her chain analysis:

1. Setting events: Lydia had a stressful day at work.

2. Trigger: Lydia's husband went to bed, and she was alone with an open bottle of wine.

3. Steps after trigger:

   a. Lydia started drinking one glass of wine.

   b. She continued to drink and finished the whole bottle.

   c. She opened another bottle and finished it, too.

4. Emotions at each point:

   a. Initially, Lydia may have felt some relief from stress while drinking.

b.  As she continued drinking, she may have felt a sense of pleasure or escape.

c.  The next morning she may have felt guilt and shame, and hungover.

5.  Intervention points:

a.  Lydia could have recognized the temptation to drink excessively and found an alternative way to cope with her stress.

b.  She could have stopped after one glass of wine and found another way to unwind before going to bed, such as journaling and reading the Bible.

c.  She could have asked for support from her husband or a friend when she felt the urge to drink more.

6.  After reviewing the chain of events and emotions that led to her drinking, Lydia explores and names the function of her behavior. She realizes that drinking helps her numb her stress and anxiety, and it provides temporary relief from negative emotions. However, she also acknowledges that her drinking behavior causes negative consequences in her life and strains her relationships.

7.  With the help of her accountability partner and licensed psychotherapist, Lydia comes up with a replacement behavior for drinking. She decides to try journaling and reading the Bible, or taking a relaxing bath after work to help her destress and cope with her emotions in a healthier way. She also sets boundaries with herself by not keeping alcohol in the house and planning to attend a support group to stay accountable. By practicing these healthier coping strategies and seeking support from others, Lydia is on her way to making positive changes in her life and strengthening her relationship with God.

In conclusion, Behavior Chain Analysis (BCA) is an effective tool for understanding and changing self-sabotaging behaviors. By breaking down a behavior into smaller components and examining setting events, triggers, thoughts, and consequences, we can identify the root causes of the behavior and develop new strategies to overcome it. It is important to identify the specific function a behavior serves and find a replacement behavior that serves the same function, but in a more positive and healthy way. Through BCA, we can gain valuable insights into our patterns of thinking and behaving, and make positive changes in our lives. As Christians, we are called to be doers of the word, and BCA can help us to break free from the cycle of self-sabotage and become more effective followers of Christ.

Dear friend, when you find yourself stuck in a pattern of self-sabotaging behavior, I want to encourage you to utilize a BCA. This technique can help you break down the chain of events leading up to the unwanted behavior and identify opportunities to intervene and make different choices. However, it is important to note that BCA is not a substitute for professional therapy or medical intervention. If you feel that your behavior is significantly impacting your life and ability to function, it is essential to seek medical help. Also, please note that alcohol detox is particularly dangerous and should never be attempted without qualified medical supervision.

It is also important to pray and ask for God's help in changing our hearts, and to seek accountability and support from trusted brothers and sisters in Christ. Do not hesitate to reach out for help if you are struggling with a particular sin or behavior. We are meant to walk together in community and encourage one another on our journey toward healing and growth.

I know that reaching out for support can be a difficult thing to do. However, I want to encourage you to contact the people on your list of safe others for assistance. It is important to remember that no one should ever judge you because we all have struggles at times, especially with the things that the Lord is working on within us.

In this journey, it is important to radically accept the Lord's love and forgiveness as you navigate through this experience. You are not alone, and God is always holding onto you even when you cannot hold onto yourself. Remember, God did not intend for us to face life alone. Even God is in community with the Holy Spirit and Jesus.

## MORE ON REPLACEMENT BEHAVIORS

As I noted earlier, to effectively conduct a Behavioral Chain Analysis, it is imperative to creatively identify replacement behaviors that can substitute for self-sabotaging behaviors. These replacement behaviors serve the same purpose as the problematic behavior, but are not harmful, are more in line with God's Word, and are more advantageous. For example, if the problematic behavior is over-using alcohol to cope with stress (i.e., the function is to escape stress/internal duress), a replacement behavior could be going for a walk, reading a favorite book, practicing Christian Diaphragmatic Breathing, or confiding in a friend. Replacement behaviors are healthy alternatives that still address the function of the original behavior.

It is important to compile a comprehensive list of replacement behaviors to use when tempted by the self-sabotaging behavior with which you struggle. Your list should include pleasurable activities consistent with your Christian value system and not lead you into more unhelpful behaviors. Here is a list of popular replacement behaviors:

1. Going for a walk in nature

2. Practicing deep breathing exercises

3. Listening to uplifting Christian music

4. Praying or meditating on Scripture

5. Reading the Bible or devotional material

6. Journaling or writing down thoughts and feelings

7. Spending time with family and friends

8. Cooking a healthy meal or trying a new recipe

9. Engaging in creative activities such as painting, drawing, or crafts

10. Exercising or trying a new physical activity

11. Volunteering or helping others in need

12. Attending church or a Bible study group

13. Gardening or spending time in nature

14. Watching an uplifting movie or show

15. Reading a book or listening to an audiobook

16. Taking a relaxing bath or shower

17. Practicing gratitude by listing blessings and positive aspects of life

18. Cleaning or organizing your living space

19. Learning a new skill or taking an online course

20. Playing a musical instrument or listening to music

21. Doing something adventurous or trying something new

22. Chewing gum or eating chocolate

23. Spending time with pets or animals

24. Dancing or participating in a group fitness class

25. Writing a letter to a loved one or friend

26. Attending a support group or seeking accountability with trusted Christian brothers or sisters

27. Worshiping the Lord

28. Reading or listening to sermons and spiritual teachings

Develop a list of pleasurable replacement activities that align with your Christian values. Creating a social media board is an effective way to keep track of them. Focus on activities that bring positive emotions, as we have noted that research shows a three-to-one positive-to-negative emotion ratio is essential for thriving. The key is to have replacements that provide the same effect as the problematic behavior. By increasing positive behaviors and removing self-sabotaging, you can more effectively enter the healing process.

## REWARDS

As you work on your *Heart Journey*™, it is important to acknowledge and celebrate your progress by rewarding yourself with positive and beneficial incentives. If shopping or spending money is not problematic, you could treat yourself by purchasing something new as a reward. For instance, if you were able to go through the month without engaging in harmful behaviors such as binging and purging (If you are struggling with binging and purging food, it is essential to seek regular therapy with a licensed psychotherapist immediately.), you could buy yourself a new blouse, outfit, or earrings as a meaningful reward. Whatever you choose as a reward, make sure it is something that brings you genuine joy and happiness.

Remember, taking care of yourself, and making progress in your journey toward healing is an accomplishment worthy of celebration. As a Christian woman, it is important to prioritize self-care and self-love, and rewarding yourself for constructive behavior is one way to do that. By taking the time to acknowledge your progress and treating yourself with a meaningful reward, you are affirming your worth and value in God's eyes.

Now it is time to go to your *Heart Journey*™ *Journal* and work through your **Eliminating Unhelpful Behaviors Heartwork.**

## CONSECRATE THE HEALING PROCESS TO THE LORD

As we continue to lay the groundwork for our heart RECONSTRUCTION™, we move into the "C," which stands for "Consecrate the Healing Process to the Lord." We want to ask the Lord into every area of this healing process. He is limitless and wants to do greater than we can ask or imagine.

When Jesus first started His public ministry, He quoted Scripture from Isaiah 61 about turning ashes into beauty. Here, the word "ashes" represents mourning. When we ask the Lord to turn our ashes into beauty, we are asking Him to transform our pain into healing.

*The Spirit of the Lord God is upon Me, Because the Lord has anointed Me to preach good tidings to the poor: He has sent Me to heal the brokenhearted ... to console those who mourn in Zion, To give them beauty for ashes, The oil of joy for mourning, The garment of praise for the spirit of heaviness; That they may be called trees of righteousness, The planting of the Lord, that He may be glorified."*

### Isaiah 61:1-3 (NKJV)

As you consecrate the healing process to the Lord, it is important to invite Him into every area of our lives and ask Him to lead us toward His will. We can start by asking Him to go into every room in our hearts and renovate according to His plan. If we struggle with doubts or lack of trust toward God, it is important to recognize that these feelings may stem from past hurts or experiences. Instead of viewing God as untrustworthy, we can lean into trust and soften into His safety, belonging, and security in our lives. By allowing God to guide the healing process, we can create a heart home filled with His love and restoration.

## LETTING HIM IN

Having your hearts and minds focused on God, along with welcoming Jesus into every area of your heart, is a great way to begin consecrating your healing process to the Lord. But are there still places where you are afraid to let Him in?

I think of the Lord waiting in the Garden of Eden during the cool of the day, while Adam and Eve frightfully hid themselves from Him after eating the forbidden fruit. In angst and longing, He sensed they were hiding from Him.

*Then the Lord called to Adam and said to him, "Where are you?"*

### Genesis 3:9 (NKJV)

God yearned for fellowship with them, did He not? And He is saying the same thing to you and me in those spaces in our heart where we are fearfully avoiding welcoming Him in. He stands at the door, knocking, yearning to come in.

I encourage you to let Him into every place in your heart. Lean in. Take some time with Him and invite Him into every area of your heart. Remember, the limitless God who created you knows exactly how to restore your heart home.

Now it is time to reopen your *Heart Journey Journal* and complete the exercise in Chapter Four, **Individual Heartwork - Consecrate to the Lord.**

## ORIENT TO RESTORATION TOOLS

As we continue with the RECONSTRUCTION™ acronym, we are going to delve into what the "O" stands for, which is "Orient to Restoration" tools.

As we prepare to move into deeper work in your heart, we now discover more emotional regulation tools that will be directly applicable to Phase Two—Deconstruction and Restoration, which begins in the next chapter.

## CHANGE AND ACCEPTANCE

The first tool you will pick up is the "Dialectic of Acceptance and Seeking Change."[14] Although this phrase may sound quite complex, it is fairly basic. "Di" means "two," and when you think about acceptance and change, they seem like opposites, but are they?

Acceptance means to accept things the way they are, without wanting anything to change. Change, on the other hand, involves moving from where we are to somewhere else. These two concepts may seem contradictory, but in reality, they complement each other. We need to accept ourselves and our circumstances, without condemning ourselves, while at the same time, pursuing change and sanctification with all our heart.

The Bible talks about the importance of both acceptance and change. In Philippians 4:11-13 (NIV), Paul writes, "I have learned to be content whatever the circumstances ... I can do all things through Him who gives me strength." This verse emphasizes the importance of finding contentment in our current situation while also striving for growth with the help of God. We are called to press on toward our goals and trust in God's strength and guidance. The Lord helps us with both acceptance and change, as He is full of mercy and lovingkindness, yet He is always growing us.

## TITRATION

The second "Orient to Restoration" tool is called "Titration."[15] It may sound complicated, but it is actually a simple concept that will help us pace ourselves through the healing journey. We will take the healing process step by step to avoid retraumatizing ourselves or overwhelming our emotions. If you ever feel like you need a break, remember to pause and use the relaxation tools we discussed earlier or reach out to a trusted person for support.

As we progress, it is crucial to stay within our Window of Tolerance, which is where your RESOURCE™ tools come in handy. We need to be mindful not to venture beyond the emotionally manageable zone and trigger our fight or flight response or dissociate. Remember, when we move out of our zone of tolerance, we lose access to our higher cortex, which makes it challenging to process information and heal effectively. Thus, we must stay within the manageable zone and use all the tools we discussed earlier to stay grounded.

The Titration process allows us to metabolize and transform trauma into healing at a manageable pace. We will explore your story and tackle difficult themes, but we will do it slowly and carefully, releasing and integrating as we go. Remember, slow and steady wins the race. We cannot force healing to happen quickly. When you plant a seed in the ground, it takes time for it to sprout and grow into a flourishing plant. Similarly, our healing journey unfolds gradually, like the blossoming of a flower. Just as rushing the growth of a plant would hinder its development, rushing our healing process can be overwhelming and counterproductive. Remember, slow is fast, and fast is overwhelming and counterproductive.

## WORK THE EDGES

"Working the Edges"[16] is another titration-informed approach that enables us to explore our traumatic experiences slowly and safely, without overwhelming our nervous system. When we experience trauma, our nervous system can go into hyperarousal or hypoarousal, which can hinder our ability to integrate our experiences and move forward. Therefore, it is crucial to work with the nervous system and gradually progress toward the traumatic event. It is important to remember that we do not heal when we bump out of the Window of Tolerance. Instead, we work from the edges into the "ground zero" of trauma, or the hardest moment of trauma, to avoid re-traumatization. As we work through trauma, we remain in God's peace and move at the pace of nervous system regulation.

Philippians 4:7 (LEB) says, "And the peace of God that surpasses all understanding will guard your hearts and your minds in Christ Jesus." This Scripture highlights that God's peace is powerful enough to guard our hearts and minds as we work through trauma. Working the Edges involves dividing the trauma into time segments and gradually working toward the heart of the trauma, T=0. We start near the edges and work our way in, building capacity for addressing the heart of the trauma as we move closer to T=0.

For example, if a dog bit you when you were younger and you are working through the trauma using *Heart Journey*™ tools for Time Reversing Trauma™, you would start with the Lord's presence and softening into His safety. Then, you would begin at T+7, when the dog bite incident was over, and you knew you had survived. Next, you would move to processing T-7, before the trauma began and when you felt safe. Then, you would process seeing the dog, followed by the dog running toward you, gradually moving into processing and discharging T=0, the actual bite. You would slowly move through T+1, screaming for help, then help coming and shooing the dog away (T+4), and finally, finish up processing when your leg was healed, and you knew it was over (T+7). In an upcoming chapter, you will learn how to process and discharge traumas as you work from the edges into the heart of trauma, but for now, it is important to familiarize yourself with the Working the Edges tool.

I did not outline all the steps of processing from T-7 to T+7 here, but we explore working the edges more in depth as we move into Time Reversing Traumas™ in Chapter Seven. Here is a graphic example of dividing a trauma up into time segments:

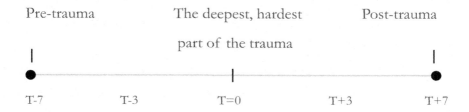

## OSCILLATION

"Oscillation" is another tool we will use in processing and resolving traumas. With this tool, we will follow an imaginary figure-eight with a stimulus on both sides, one highly positive and one negative and associated with a trauma. We will use our holy imaginations to oscillate along the figure-eight to integrate the negative with the positive, using a mechanism in our brain that is called Memory Reconsolidation.

Scientists believe that Memory Reconsolidation is a process by which the emotional portion of memories can be modified and updated with new emotional learning. We will learn more about Memory Reconsolidation in Chapter Six. The process involves the retrieval of a memory, followed by its destabilization and restabilization. During the destabilization phase, the memory becomes labile and susceptible to change.[17] This is where the figure-eight Oscillation technique comes in. The technique involves opening up the trauma memory with the negative stimulus and simultaneously creating a prediction error with the positive stimulus. By oscillating back and forth between the positive and negative stimuli, we can facilitate the integration of new, positive emotional learning into the memory and reduce the emotional distress associated with it.

When we use the Oscillation tool, we imagine an invisible three-foot figure-eight in the air right in front of you, positioned horizontally, so that the loops are facing left and right. The two sides of the figure-eight represent different experiences for you, and we will trace the figure-eight with our attention and imagination. While tracing the right loop, you will think about a highly positive image, and when you are tracing the left loop, you will think about the trigger you want to defuse. We are constantly mindful of the need to stay within a manageable emotional zone, the Window of Tolerance. We will continue to loop around over and over through the figure-eight until our emotions stabilize, even when we are working with the negative stimulus.

We start out spending much less time on the left side (the trigger), and we spend more time on the right (the positive). We tune into how our body feels as we are exposed to both sides of the Oscillation (the trigger and the highly positive stimulus). By doing so, we gradually gain a tolerance for expanding our time in the left side (with the trigger) as the trigger loses negative emotional valence. Practicing Oscillation will slowly discharge and reconsolidate the trigger as we trace this figure-eight in our imaginations.

As an example, let us consider Katelyn who is afraid of dogs after experiencing a vicious dog bite in third grade. The memory of the dog bite is highly triggering for Katelyn and overwhelms her, pushing her out of her Window of Tolerance. However, Katelyn wants to release this painful memory and no longer feel terrified of dogs. In our teaching example, we use the memory of the dog bite as the negative trigger (left loop) and Katelyn's grandmother's cookie jar as a highly positive memory and image for the right loop.

By using Oscillation, Katelyn unlocks the power of Memory Re-consolidation in her mind, which changes her emotional learning about dogs and helps discharge the underlying trauma. As Katelyn oscillates repeatedly through the imaginary figure-eight, between a small amount of exposure to the dog bite and a significant amount of exposure to Grandma's cookie jar, her emotions about the dog bite begin to stabilize, and she feels better. After oscillating for several minutes, with increasing exposure to the left/trigger side, Katelyn experiences a sense of stability, as if the dog bite is being defused by the happy memory.

Here is a visual representation:

If the trigger on the left side of the oscillation is too intense, we can start with a less triggering image, such as a picture of a toy poodle, and gradually work up to the actual memory of the dog bite, using the Titration tool in conjunction with the Oscillation tool.

## OVER- AND UNDER-COUPLING[18]

When we experience trauma or challenges, it is common for things to become over-coupled or under-coupled in our emotional experiences. Take Erica, for example, who was abused by her father, yet he was also a protective parental figure and advocate when she was bullied in the neighborhood. Erica feels confused because she has a "good dad" and also a "not-so-good dad" all mixed up into an overall sense of confusion about her father. It can be helpful to uncouple the good dad from the bad dad by processing each "dad" separately. This allows Erica to make sense of her history and be able to metabolize both sides of her emotions.

Although this may seem unusual to process each "dad" separately, the over-coupling of the "dads" creates serious emotional confusion that results in a double bind. Erica cannot allow herself to feel angry at her dad because she remembers the "good dad." She also cannot feel happy about her father because she remembers his abuse. She is baffled and stuck.

Over-coupling can create serious emotional confusion and result an emotional double bind. Just like Pavlov's dogs learned that the bell was tied to food, trauma can be tied to certain stimuli. For instance, someone who has been in a car accident may have over-coupled driving with survival responses like the fear of dying. It is important to be able to drive safely without feeling like we are in a life or death situation every time we get behind the wheel.

On the other hand, sometimes memories can be under-coupled. For example, after a car accident, we may not have access to any feelings about the tragic event, leaving us feeling numb. However, we may experience nausea every time we get into a car. In order to heal, we need to connect the nausea feelings to the accident, process them, and integrate them from a nervous system perspective. Essentially, our feelings need to be recoupled.

## MIRROR NEURONS AND SUPPORT

Earlier in our study, we emphasized the significance of social support. Mirror neurons, a type of brain cell, become active both during the performance of an action and when observing someone else performing the same action. They facilitate empathy, imitation, and social learning.

According to researchers, mirror neurons are thought to have a key role in social co-regulation, enabling individuals to comprehend and harmonize with the emotional and behavioral states of others, thus promoting interpersonal bonding and social unity. For instance, when we witness someone smiling, our mirror neurons activate, inducing a similar emotional response, allowing us to feel empathy and sense the emotions of others. The ability to co-regulate with others through the activation of mirror neurons is critical in building healthy relationships and supporting our healing journey.

When we are in a safe and supportive environment, our mirror neurons can be activated in a positive way, which can help us feel more secure, connected, and supported. Conversely, if we are in an unsafe or unsupportive environment, our mirror neurons can be activated in a negative way, leading to feelings of anxiety, fear, and isolation. It is a testament to the wonderful design of our Creator that we are built-in with the ability to co-regulate with each other through the activation of mirror neurons.

Therefore, Beloved, it is important to remember that building and maintaining healthy relationships and having a supportive community is vital for our well-being. This is not optional; we require a supportive community to navigate difficult experiences and promote healing. We need to surround ourselves with people who love us, support us, and help us feel safe so our mirror neurons can be activated in a positive way, and we can experience the full benefits of co-regulation.

Take time now to go to your *Heart Journey*™ *Journal* to Chapter Four and complete the **Individual Heartwork - Orient to Reconstruction Tools, Individual Heartwork - Healthy Behaviors,** and the **Heart Group Discussion - Time to Share.**

## REVIEW OF TOOLS

As we wrap up this chapter before going deeper, take some time to review the tools we have learned. If you are in a small group, you may want to discuss the different tools and learn how others are utilizing them for healing. Also, if you are unsure how or when to use them, take this time to seek and listen to the experiences of your sisters in Christ.

Friend, I am excited because you now are loaded with tools! As we are about to move into the deeper Heartwork, let us review our list of Stability tools!

1. Reframe by Inventorying Your Thinking

2. Reframe through Mind Mansion™

3. Reframe through Daily Journal Practice

4. Enrich with Positive Memories

5. Uncoupling Exercise

6. Enrich with Safe Place Imagery

7. Enrich with Eyes of Jesus™

8. Structure Your Life: Self-Care

9. Structure Your Life: Life Edit

10. Structure Your Life: Seven Types of Rest

11. Occupy the Body: Grounding

12. Occupy the Body: Body Soothing

13. Occupy the Body: Tracking

14. Undergird with Support: Identify Safe People

15. Undergird with Support: Socialgram™

16. Relaxation Skills: Christian Progressive Relaxation

17. Relaxation Skills: Christian Diaphragmatic Breathing

18. Relaxation Skills: Christian Four Square Breathing

19. Relaxation Skills: Christian Body Scan

20. Relaxation Skills: 5, 4, 3, 2, 1 Meditation-Christian Version

21. Comfort through Self-Momming™!

22. Enlighten with Content

23. Change and Acceptance

24. Oscillation

25. Titration

Before moving on to the next section, it is important to ensure you are in a safe and supportive environment that helps you feel grounded. This will help you fully engage with the upcoming work and make the most of this transformative experience.

I am thrilled to share that in the next section, we will begin to rewrite the narrative the enemy may have imposed on you. Together, we will explore and embrace the narrative God has designed for your life. I cannot wait to embark on this next phase of our journey with you.

## LET US PRAY.

*Heavenly Father,*

*Thank You for being with us on this journey. Delving into matters of the heart can get messy, but we know Your son, Jesus, is a master at transforming our messes into beautiful messages. Father, may we continue to focus on You during this process, staying ever so close to You. Lord, if our hearts and minds wander and we get off course, please gently set us back on the path to healing as only You can do.*

*In Jesus' name, Amen.*

# *Chapter*

## FIVE

### Restoring My Narrative

*And the God of all grace, who called you to His eternal glory in Christ,
after you have suffered a little while, will Himself restore you and make
you strong, firm and steadfast.*

**I Peter 5:10 (NIV)**

Have you ever desired to become the protagonist of a novel, filled with unexpected twists and turns in an enthralling plot, ultimately emerging victorious over all adversities while discovering true life-long love? While it may seem implausible at this stage of your journey, we have reached a juncture where we commence the procedures of rewriting your story, leading you toward healing, and affectionate encounters with Jesus. And I could not be prouder of you for your labors to get to this point. Give yourself a big hug, and then, with steely determination, let us delve into narrating your story.

In this chapter, we embark on a profound journey of self-discovery as we explore the power of "N" in our RECONSTRUCTION™ acronym: Narrate Your Story™. Together, we will courageously explore the intricate tapestry of our personal histories, uncovering the deceptive narratives and relentless lies the enemy has woven into our lives, attempting to hinder us from walking in our divine destiny. But fear not, for the truth remains steadfast—our God is greater than any defamation or falsehood. Now is the time, Beloved, to reclaim our narrative and rewrite it according to the magnificent plans God has ordained for us. Can you fathom the immense grace? It may seem too extraordinary to grasp, but rest assured, it is true. Our Heavenly Father longs to bestow upon us the absolute finest, intricately fashioning a purposeful life that embraces our unique qualities, even weaving our imperfections, challenges, and stumbling blocks into the masterpiece of our journey (Psalm 139:16).

## SAFETY FIRST

At this point in your journey, if you are not feeling safe, wanting to engage in self-harming behaviors, feeling like your life is still too out of control, or you are perpetually overwhelmed, go back to your RESOURCE™ tools. Keep practicing these tools until your nervous system is more regulated and ready for looking at your history. And remember, it is always a good option to see a licensed psychotherapist. Many psychotherapist search databases have options for searching for a "Christian" licensed psychotherapist, if so desired.

For those of you who are ready, we will begin with a few strategies to utilize as needed to reduce emotional overwhelm while we go through constructing our narrative.

## DISTANCING STRATEGIES

As we work through the next three chapters, you will, at times, need to use Distancing Strategies, which can be helpful when we experience overwhelming memory content and need to apply emotional distance to stay regulated in our nervous system.

## BINOCULARS BACKWARDS™

Our first strategy is "Binoculars Backwards™." When used properly, binoculars zoom in on what is observed. But flipped backwards, the view zooms out to give us space from what we observe. Remember, we want to stay within the Window of Tolerance, so when we are accessing a painful memory and we feel over-activated or like we want to dissociate, we can zoom out with Binoculars Backwards™. Dissociation is a psychological state in which we experience a detachment or disconnection from our surroundings, thoughts, feelings, or sense of self, often resulting in a sense of numbness or emotional distance. If you bump into fight or flight or freeze, or down into depression, numbness, dissociation, feeling floaty, or your mind goes blank, you are likely outside of a Window of Tolerance. The aim of *Heart Journey*™ is not to retraumatize you, and effective Memory Reconsolidation happens within the Window of Tolerance. Therefore, we want to get some space by thinking about content from a distance, as needed. Binoculars Backwards™ helps us regulate by mentally zooming out from the pain to a bird's eye view.

## MOVIE SCREEN STRATEGY

Another Distancing tool is the "Movie Screen Strategy," which involves visualizing or imagining the painful memory content is displayed on a movie screen. This approach provides a regulating sense of detachment since the screen is external to you, allowing you to create some distance from the content. To increase this effect, you can even sit at the back of the cinema while reviewing your memories.

## "IT'S OVER" STRATEGY

Our third technique is known as the "It's Over" Strategy. When we encounter a distressing memory, we can remind ourselves that the event has concluded. We recall when we recognized it was over, that is when we felt relieved the situation had ended. We courageously assure our inner child that the scene has passed, and we are currently safe. The painful experiences and unmet needs from our childhood or adulthood are in the past. Allow that fact to permeate your being. At times, it is helpful to remember when we experienced that sense of relief, that "Aah! It's over." When this tool applies, soften into that relief sensation. You might even want to repeat out loud: "It's over. I survived, and God is going to turn my ashes into beauty."

## RESOURCE™ AND ENJOY THE JOURNEY

Make sure to utilize the RESOURCE™ tools throughout the continuation of this study, as they will assist in creating a sense of safety and security. When we renovate a house, we always prioritize safety and stability. We work on one part of the house at a time to ensure functionality for those who live in the house. Similarly, we want you to remain functional, so if you ever feel overwhelmed, it is time to take a break. Engage in pleasurable activities like spending time with friends. Step away from your *Heart Journey*™ work and give yourself a pause, then come back to it as you are ready. Remember to enjoy the journey and embrace laughter as a crucial component of your healing. We move at the pace of grace.

## HEAL WITH OTHERS

Beloved, I strongly advise working through this chapter, as well as the next three chapters of this study, with a trusted friend, counselor, or licensed psychotherapist if you are not in a small group. This chapter will involve writing, drawing, creating a timeline, and journaling about your history. I encourage you to share your entries with at least one safe individual who can pray with you and support you throughout this process—someone who comprehends the journey and may have even navigated their own.

## TIMELINE WORK

At this step, "Narrate Your Story™," we are moving beyond stabilization and diving into the heart of restoration work, which involves delving into our past experiences. It is important to do so because our past wounds often create the areas of emotional gridlock in our current lives.

For instance, Felicia grew up with an emotionally distant and critical father. This led to a pattern of seeking approval from men and feeling unworthy and unlovable. She struggles with trusting others and often sabotages her relationships, fearing she will be rejected or abandoned.

Allison grew up in a family where painful emotions were not validated, and toxic positivity was the norm. Toxic positivity refers to the harmful and excessive promotion of positive thinking and feeling, denying or invalidating genuine negative emotions and experiences, which can lead to emotional suppression and lack of authentic support. As a result, she developed a pattern of denying and suppressing her own painful emotions, which led to difficulties in expressing herself and connecting with others in her adult life.

While your story may differ from Felicia's or Allison's, the past is likely impacting your present in some way. That is why it is important to follow the steps outlined in this chapter to "Narrate Your Story™," so you can begin the process of healing. However, since we will be working with painful memories in the upcoming chapters, it is essential to take your time with this deeper work and remember to titrate.

"Timeline work" is a powerful tool in the heart healing process, allowing us to identify and address the positive and negative events that have impacted our lives. Research has shown that narrative work can be effective in treating depression, anxiety, and trauma.[19] "Narrate Your Story™" involves creating timelines of different ages throughout our life, pinpointing hurts, wounds, unmet needs, and positive events that have left an impression on the heart. By looking at these events in a structured way, we will begin to identify patterns and themes that have developed in our lives, both positive and negative. This process can help to enhance the positive aspects of our history while also identifying our targets, that is trauma and unmet needs, for reconstruction.

As believers, we can find encouragement in Scripture as we undertake the work of healing our hearts. The woman at the well, known as the Samaritan woman, had a difficult past and was struggling with her reputation in her community when she met Jesus. However, Jesus saw beyond her hurt and pain, and helped her see herself in a new narrative. He encouraged her to find identity in Him as His cherished child, instead of being defined by her excruciating past. This encounter caused the Samaritan woman to develop into a woman of purpose. She left a lasting legacy that is still remembered today. You, too, have a great legacy before you, but you must face the past and allow the finger of God to rewrite its imprint on your heart.

## INTRODUCTION TO NARRATIVE WORK

Beloved, we are going to create timelines of different ages through-out your life and pinpoint the hurts, wounds, unmet needs, and positive events that have impacted you. Your timeline work will be the basis of our healing encounters over the next three chapters. We are about to discover the positive and negative events that have impacted your life, thoughts and beliefs about yourself and your inner world. We will also look for themes that God has developed through your life, and themes the enemy has tried to watermark upon your life. God is truth and the enemy is a liar. We want to amalgamate our beliefs about ourselves with our Creator's truth, and thereby find lavish belonging and fulfilling purpose.

We will be creating several timelines, exploring the keystone experiences within your early childhood, elementary school years, middle school years, high school years, young adulthood, and adulthood. For each of these timelines, we will be identifying all the impactful events, whether positive or negative, that have shaped your heart and impacted your life. Our goal is to retain the positive and allow Jesus to transform the negative events that have wounded you. Beloved, all your work will be worth it! Our narrative work through timelines is laying the foundation for the work ahead.

## PRACTICE IMPERFECTIONISM

We will embrace imperfectionism, recognizing that striving for perfect timelines can lead to overwhelming pressure and fear of falling short, ultimately immobilizing our progress. While it is important to not skip any steps, I ask that you give up perfectionism and complete what you can reasonably manage. Trust that God is at work in your heart home and will address all the areas that need recovery.

Furthermore, it is important to note that you can revisit this study as many times as you need. What is important is that you continue to take steps forward. Consistency is more important than perfection, as my workout coach reminds me, and we have a powerful and loving God with us every step of the way. We can do this! You can do this!

# TIMELINE WORK

Let us forge ahead and ascend to new heights as we chart our personal histories, pinpoint pivotal moments, and explore emerging themes. Refer to your *Heart Journey*™ *Journal* **Individual Heartwork - Narrate Your Story**™ **Activity,** where you will construct timelines for various stages of your life, starting with ages zero through five, and continuing with each subsequent timeline. It is crucial to identify positive events, as well as any traumas and unmet needs associated with each timeline. Although we will begin with the timeline for ages zero to five, the process will remain the same for each subsequent timeline. Remember to label your timeline with positive events, as well as any traumas or unmet needs.

Here are the steps you will employ for each timeline:

1. Write the formative positive experiences that occurred in the designated age range on top of the timeline at the ages these experiences occurred.

2. Write the formative negative, wounding, traumatizing, and/ or painful experiences that occurred in that age range on the bottom of the timeline at the ages these experiences occurred. Keep in mind that perception is fundamental in trauma work, and it is important not to judge whether an event "should" be included at the bottom of your timeline. If you feel like it is relevant, then it is worth listing. Do not hesitate to include events from both family and non-family settings, as they all play a role in shaping our experiences.

3. Use colored pencils or markers to label events on the bottom of your timeline as traumas ("T") or unmet needs ("UN").

4. After all your timelines are completed, you will then look for themes throughout your life, both positive and negative. Positive themes are written down within your life from the

Lord, and negative themes have been seeded by the enemy. Sample themes include:

a. Defectiveness vs. acceptance (e.g., I am bad; I am accepted)

b. Unsafe vs. safe (e.g., I am not safe; I am safe)

c. Difficulty with trust vs. trust (e.g., I cannot trust; I can trust)

d. Feeling no power/ no control vs. power (e.g., I am powerless; My voice matters)

e. Not belonging vs. belonging (e.g., I do not belong; I belong)

f. Not feeling connected vs. feeling connected (e.g., I am alone vs I am connected)

## MEMORY AND DEVELOPMENT

It is important to keep in mind when working on your timeline for ages zero to five, you may not have many memories from before the age of three. This is a normal occurrence, as our autobiographical memory typically begins to develop around the age of three when expressive language strongly emerges. Furthermore, our brains undergo significant pruning and reorganization through the age of seven, which can result in natural memory loss. During this age range, it is often common for individuals to have fragmented recollections of events, relying on stories passed down, photographs, or retaining only a select few memories. Therefore, it is possible you may not have as much information for this timeline. Looking at pictures or interviewing family members may be helpful for jogging your early memory.

## TRAUMA AND MEMORY LOSS

Research has shown that some individuals who have experienced trauma may have sparse memories due to the impact of stress on the brain. However, with the help of regulating the nervous system through the use of RESOURCE™ skills, memories can slowly resurface. It is crucial to recognize that memories should not be coerced or forcefully unearthed, but rather allowed to resurface naturally. The tools provided in this and the following chapters can aid in working with existing memories, potentially helping other memories to resurface. In addition, as one progresses through the *Heart Journey*™ process, emotions and memories that were previously frozen can thaw, allowing for the emergence of more positive memories and emotions.[20]

Just as our physical bodies have a natural healing process, so do our hearts. It is important to trust in this process and not force memories to come to the surface before we are ready. Our hearts may have developed dissociation as a coping mechanism to protect us from overwhelming emotions and memories. Therefore, we must be gentle with ourselves and allow memories to come forth naturally as we progress through the *Heart Journey*™. If too many memories are surfacing and causing us to feel overwhelmed, we can slow down the process and use our Distancing Strategies and RESOURCE™ skills to regulate our nervous system.

## ZERO TO FIVE TIMELINE

Now for our timeline work! We will devote extra attention to elaborating on the process of creating your zero to five timeline as an example to help guide you for all your timeline work. On the top of your timeline, list the formative positive experiences that occurred in this age range. On the bottom, list the negative events that occurred. We want to capture the highlights of this age range where your need for love, safety, and belonging were met and you were celebrated, as well as the traumas and unmet needs from your history.

## SURFACE-LEVEL EXPLORATION

As you work through the Heartwork in this chapter, try to avoid emotionally immersing yourself in every memory. Instead, focus on identifying and recording memories while remaining in a more surface-level zone. To illustrate this point, I often tell my clients, "Think of it like looking at a map of your life. We do not need to travel to every city and experience every memory right now." It is important to maintain some distance to avoid becoming overwhelmed by your entire timeline. We will delve into individual memories explicitly in a titrated manner later on.

## TRAUMAS

The Bible does not use the term "trauma" directly, but it describes events that could be considered traumatic, such as war, natural disasters, and interpersonal violence. In Psalm 34:18 (NIV), it says, "The LORD is close to the brokenhearted and saves those who are crushed in spirit." This verse acknowledges the pain of those who are experiencing deep emotional distress. In Isaiah 61:1 (NIV), it says, "The Spirit of the Sovereign LORD is on me because the LORD has anointed me to proclaim good news to the poor. He has sent me to bind up the brokenhearted, to proclaim freedom for the captives and release from darkness for the prisoners." This verse acknowledges that people can be brokenhearted and captive to their circumstances, but God can bring healing and freedom. Additionally, in Psalm 147:3 (NKJV), it says, "He heals the brokenhearted and binds up their wounds." This verse implies that God can bring healing to emotional wounds, just as He can heal physical wounds. These verses demonstrate that the Bible acknowledges the reality of trauma and the need for healing from it.

Trauma can be defined as a deeply distressing or disturbing experience that overwhelms our ability to cope and negatively impacts our emotional and psychological well-being. Trauma occurs when our sense of safety is shattered and can result from a variety of experiences. Other ways to define trauma include the following:

1. experiencing too much too soon, such as sexual experiences in childhood or being forced to take on a parental role as a child;

2. enduring too little for too long, such as insufficient food, safety, or belonging;

3. facing too much too quickly, such as a sudden and overwhelming painful experience that leaves us no time to process, such as being trapped in an avalanche;

4. suffering too much for too long, such as ongoing verbal abuse from a parent or bully; or,

5. experiencing too much with too little support, such as going through difficult circumstances, like war, without anyone to process and validate our feelings.

Dear one, trauma can come in many forms and can vary greatly from person to person. It is important to remember that trauma is a personal and subjective experience, and each individual will have their own unique experiences and reactions. Nonetheless, here is a list of some traumas that women have experienced themselves, or within their families, to help get you thinking about your own experiences. Remember, these events might be experienced as traumatic if they happen to you, or if you experience trauma vicariously. Vicarious trauma refers to the emotional and psychological impact experienced by individuals who are indirectly exposed to the trauma of others, such as through hearing their stories or witnessing their suffering, leading to similar symptoms and distress as those directly affected by the trauma. In addition, witnessing trauma can have a traumatic impact.

Abandonment

Abuse (physical, emotional, sexual)

Accidents

Addiction

Attack (by animal or person)

Betrayal

Bullying

Cancer

Car crashes

Childhood neglect

Chronic illness

Combat trauma

Death of a loved one

Divorce

Domestic violence

Emotional neglect

Financial loss

Fire

Forced displacement

Foster care system

Home invasion

House fire

Near choking

Near death experience

Near drowning

Parental incarceration

Physical illness

Physical neglect

Police brutality

Political violence

Poisoning

Poverty

Racism

Rape

Refugee trauma

Religious trauma

School shootings

Sexual harassment

Sibling abuse

Social isolation

Stalking

Substance abuse in the family

Suicide of a loved one

Terrorist attacks

Immigration trauma                 Torture

Infertility                        Traumatic injury

Job loss                           War

Kidnapping                         Workplace harassment

Medical trauma

Miscarriage

Natural disasters

As you work on creating your trauma inventory, it is crucial to honor and acknowledge your own experience. Pay attention to your emotions and reactions as you go through the process of creating your inventory, and do not hesitate to include events that may not have been listed but still had a significant impact on you. This includes any prenatal traumatic events during your zero to five timeline, such as if your mother was assaulted while you were in utero. Although we may not have autobiographical memory during our early years, our bodies have implicit memory where traumas can be held, even prenatally. Witnessing domestic violence or any type of violence is also considered traumatic for children. Marginalized populations may experience traumatic macro- and micro-aggressions due to prejudiced attitudes and behaviors. All of these experiences are traumatic and should be included on our timelines. Traumas are like "sins" of commission that happen to us, while unmet needs are "sins" of omission where our deepest God-given needs are not met, whether deliberately or not.

## UNMET NEEDS

Scripture and psychology—separately and together—help us as Christians (or other people of faith) understand our unmet needs. From a psychological perspective, our needs are fundamental aspects of our well-being that must be met in order for us to develop in a healthy trajectory. These needs can be physical, emotional, spiritual, relational, or related to safety and nourishment. When our early needs are not met, it can lead to a variety of psychological issues and negative relationship outcomes.

The Bible emphasizes the importance of positive experiences and parenting for children. Proverbs 22:6 (ESV) says, "Train up a child in the way he should go; even when he is old he will not depart from it." This shows the importance of providing children with a positive and nurturing environment in which they can grow and develop. Similarly, Ephesians 6:4 instructs fathers to not provoke their children to anger, but to bring them up in the discipline and instruction of the Lord. This emphasizes the importance of providing children with guidance and direction grounded in love and patience.

Jesus also exemplified the importance of valuing and treating children with love and care. In Mark 10:13-16 (ESV), Jesus said, "Let the little children come to me, and do not hinder them, for the kingdom of God belongs to such as these." He welcomed and blessed the children, demonstrating that they are valuable and loved in the eyes of God.

Additionally, in Matthew 18:5 (AMP), Jesus said, "Whoever receives one such child in My name receives Me." This further emphasizes the importance of showing love and care to children. Overall, these Scriptures demonstrate the significance of meeting childhood needs so children develop into healthy and well-rounded individuals.

When taking an inventory of your unmet needs, it is important to examine how your physical, emotional, spiritual, attachment, relational, safety, and nourishment needs were met or not met. It is also valuable to consider whether your need for appropriate discipline was met or not. For example, were you given appropriate consequences when you misbehaved? Did your parents provide structure and guidance in a loving and validating environment? Research shows that children who thrive have parents who provide warmth, love, validation, and security, as well as structure and boundaries. Consider taking the time to reflect on your childhood experiences and even speaking with a family member to gain more insight into your needs and how they were met.

## DEVELOPMENTAL NEEDS AND STAGES OF LIFE

Regardless of the stage of life we find ourselves in, the need for validation of our identity and the desire to be heard, understood, and accepted remains constant. In addition, some of our needs evolve with experience, and new needs emerge developmentally. Below is a summary of many of our psychological needs as we grow from early childhood into adulthood. Although spiritual needs are not heavily addressed below, we certainly have spiritual needs, and I encourage you to put those on your timeline. From a Christian worldview, we would want to be introduced to Christ at a young age, and be taught His word, His grace, His truth, and His ways. We want to know Him at each age and stage. Identify what needs were met and not met as you read through the below summary.

**Zero to Five.** In the first five years of life, our brains and emotional centers are rapidly developing. As such, our primary need is for consistent and responsive caregiving from our parents or guardians. It is essential to be in environments where we feel safe, and our needs for nourishment, love, and supervision are met. We require a secure base in at least one parent to develop autonomy and the ability to explore with boundaries. Validation of our individuality is crucial, and we need room for emotional expression, so we feel enjoyed and validated for who we are.

**Elementary School Years.** The elementary school years, typically between ages five to ten, is a period of intense learning and growth. During this time, we become increasingly independent and industrious. As we navigate the complexities of school and peer relationships, we need the support and validation of our parents to guide us through emotional challenges and provide us with structure and guidance. We also require a sense of belonging both at home and in school, which helps us feel secure and nurtured. As we begin to discover our unique interests and hobbies, we develop a deeper understanding of how God has created us and our place in the world.

**Middle School Years.** The middle school years can be tumultuous and challenging, as we grapple with many issues of identity and self-discovery. As we navigate these years, usually between the ages of eleven to thirteen, we rely on our parents to provide a safe and secure base, while giving us just the right amount of autonomy and parenting. It is essential to have validation and support as we develop our sense of self and purpose. Parents play a critical role in providing guidance and structure, helping us navigate peer relationships, and creating opportunities for growth and development. It is important to remember that some tension between us and our parents is natural during this time, but it is essential to maintain a high level of love and structure to help us navigate these challenging years.

**High School Years**. As we enter high school, typically between the ages of fourteen and eighteen, we are on a fast track toward adulthood. We continue to need validation, belonging, space for our emotions, guidance, and structure, but we are given more autonomy. Our parents gradually shift into the role of consultants, preparing us for the independence we will have in adulthood. During this time, our peer group becomes increasingly important, and we need to feel a sense of belonging and acceptance within it. We also need opportunities to explore and develop our interests and talents, as well as support in planning and preparing for our future.

**Young Adulthood.** In young adulthood, we are exploring the world and discovering our place in it. We need positive peer groups that help us develop in the areas of career, relationships, and adulthood. We benefit from having mentors who can guide us and provide us with insight and wisdom as we make important life decisions. As we embark on new adventures, we still need a sense of belonging and validation from our family and loved ones. Our parents can serve as older and wiser advisors, offering support and guidance as we navigate through the challenges of young adulthood. They can help us develop a stronger sense of identity, and provide us with a safe haven to return to when we need support and encouragement. At the same time, young adulthood is a time of exploration and self-discovery, and we need the freedom to make our own decisions and take responsibility for our own lives. As we take steps toward independence, it is important to remember we still need love, guidance, and support from the people in our lives who have our best interests at heart.

**Adulthood.** In adulthood, one of our primary needs is to establish safe and fulfilling relationships with our peers, family, and possibly our significant other. We need people who can support us emotionally, who can communicate effectively, and who can help us navigate through the challenges life brings. We need to come to terms with our sexual self. In terms of our career or ministry, we need to develop our skills and expertise in order to make a meaningful impact in the world through living out our God-given purpose. We need to master practical, social, and love domains, which include financial management, social skills, and healthy relationships. Finally, as we grow older, we need to think about the legacy we want to leave behind for future generations.

## TWO LIFE ASSIGNMENTS

In life, God has a unique purpose for each one of us (Jeremiah 29:11). He writes good themes of love, belonging, discipline, and unique purpose into our stories (Ephesians 2:10). In fact, He has written a whole book of purpose about us (Psalm 139:16)! However, we must also recognize the enemy is always trying to write a counter assignment over us, full of death and rejection (John 10:10).

As we discover negative themes around defectiveness, safety, vulnerability, power, and control, it is important to remember these motifs depict the enemy's counter assignment for us. These lies are not what God wants for us, and it is our goal to fight against them with the powerful Word of God.

The enemy may try to write themes like, "there is something wrong with me," "I deserve bad things to happen," "I have to be perfect to be loved," "It is all my fault," "I cannot trust anyone," "I am powerless to get what I need," "I am a failure," or "I cannot handle it." These are common themes for those who have experienced developmental trauma or unmet needs in childhood.

But despite what the enemy has been trying to write into your life, we can destroy those words with the truth of God's Word (Hebrews 4:12). His word is powerful and active, able to divide soul and spirit. The Lord is more than able to transform us from the inside out with His word.

We will heal as we renew our minds with the Scriptures that speak to our specific struggles (Romans 12:2). It is important to pray for insight over what themes the Lord wants to write into our lives and allow the truth of God's Word to simmer and marinate within our hearts, producing transformation. God wants to turn our ashes into beauty (Isaiah 61:3). He wants to pour out His Spirit and set our captive hearts free (Luke 4:18-19). And He wants us to transform into our true selves, the opposite of what the enemy tried to write into us.

Now it is time for you to look over your traumas and unmet needs, as well as the positive events that have occurred in your life, and deeply drink in the themes God has been imprinting upon you, casting off the themes the enemy has been attempting to imprint upon you. You will counter the lies of the enemy with Scripture. This is an important part of your work. You can find your own Scriptures to specifically counter the lies of the enemy, or you can use sample Scriptures that are helpful in regard to understanding your identity in Christ and are listed in your

*Heart Journey*™ *Journal.* Use His Scripture like medicine, meditate on it several times a day, and let it become your new identity as the favored child of God, the theme of your life (Psalm 1:1-3).

## RESPONSIBILITY PIE CHART

In your Heartwork found in your *Heart Journey*™ *Journal,* you will also create a Responsibility Pie Chart. Responsibility Pie Charts are merely pie charts that show who is culpable for certain events in our history. Sometimes, we share a percentage of culpability regarding the occurrence of a series of events, but what can end up happening is that we errantly take responsibility for the full event because we shared partial responsibility. In other words, we allow "false guilt."

## FALSE GUILT

False guilt is a type of guilt that arises from a belief that one has done something wrong or bad, even though there is no actual evidence or reason to support this belief. False guilt is often rooted in the lies of the enemy and can keep us from experiencing the freedom and joy that God intends for us (John 8:44). False guilt is not from God and can lead to negative emotions such as shame, anxiety, and despair. It is important to distinguish false guilt from true guilt, which arises from a genuine recognition of one's own wrongdoing or sin.

An example of an appropriate use of a Responsibility Pie Chart might be in the case of a teenage girl who lied to her parents and snuck out in the middle of the night to meet a boy. Sadly, she was assaulted by the boy, and ended up feeling like the entire assault was her fault because she snuck out. In truth, when we chart the event, the perpetrator is entirely responsible for the assault; however, the teenage girl shares a piece of responsibility in the overall culpability in the series of events in that she disobeyed and deceived her parents by sneaking out. She is responsible for the lying but not the assault. Here, we can use two pie charts. On one, we would identify that the perpetrator is 100 percent responsible for the assault, and on the other, we identify that the teenage girl is 100 percent responsible for the deception. The teenage girl is zero percent responsible for the assault. Employing the Responsibility Pie Chart relieves our consciousness from false guilt, and empowers us to repent over true guilt. We must shake the dust off our feet in regard to false guilt. Beloved, condemnation does not belong to us. Regarding true guilt, we will work on forgiveness in a later chapter.

## BACK TO DEBORAH'S STORY

Our friend Deborah whom you met previously, gained valuable insights as she worked on her timelines. All these insights prepared her for the encounters she would have with Jesus in the next steps in her *Heart Journey*™.

Deborah rediscovered that dance had played a significant role in her life from childhood through her mid-teens. Deborah found a strong sense of belonging through dance, as her friends were involved, and her family frequently took her to dance classes. It surprised her that she had forgotten how important dance had been until she completed her timeline work. It seemed as if the losses in her life had blocked her ability to remember the good moments.

In addition, Deborah identified several traumas she added to her timelines. For example, she recorded the day when her mother slapped her violently in front of a visiting friend. This incident not only scared her friend, but it also embarrassed Deborah. Prior to this event, Deborah had always felt lonely, as she had never connected with her mother while growing up, increasing the pain of this event.

Deborah identified many themes, including several that arose from her mother's constant criticism about her weight. Her mother frequently attempted to place Deborah on a diet, and this developed into a fear of not having enough food as well as shame about her body.

Deborah acknowledged the fear and shame as recurring themes the enemy had written into her life. As early as elementary school, Deborah began using food as a coping mechanism. Psychologically isolated, Deborah felt neglected, was bullied, and witnessed domestic violence, which all established an insecure base and themes of rejection and insecurity. This all fed into her struggles with emotional eating. Taken together, Deborah discovered recurring themes throughout her life that included food scarcity, body shame, and feeling unsafe, alone, unimportant, and insignificant both in her family and in school.

## RENOUNCING AND CHOOSING BELIEFS

Speaking truth in the face of lies planted by the enemy is indispensable in changing the atmosphere that defines our inner lives. In your Heartwork, you will renounce lies and speak the truth where you discover deception in your timeline work. After searching the Scriptures, we can find specific passages to combat the lies the enemy has tried to engrave into our minds.

We can also use our Reframing tool on our themes. Scroll back to our Inventory Your Thinking tool from RESOURCE™ and review our list of thinking errors. Inspect your themes for thinking errors that you can turn around using Inventory Your Thinking tool. Deborah's timeline work included themes of defectiveness. She often felt defective and worthy of rejection even though she loathed the experience of rejection. She used the Inventory Your Thinking tool on demonically inspired rejection themes in her timeline, and stated, "Now I know I am fearfully and wonderfully made and desirable because of how God made me."

## EMOTIONS

Beloved, you are familiar with my encouragement to stay within the Window of Tolerance and to utilize your RESOURCE™ skills. However, it is important to recognize that difficult emotions will arise as you work through your timelines. To address the underlying issues causing you to feel stuck, it is impossible to avoid experiencing challenging emotions. Despite this, I want to remind you that there is hope at the end of the tunnel.

In the upcoming chapters, we will be facing some difficult themes and emotions, but it is necessary to address our wounds and pain to find freedom. As you go through this process, remember to rely on your sisters, the Lord, and to make time for recreation and enjoyment. It is important to maintain a balance between feeling the emotions of your life and enjoying your life. Do not succumb to the temptation of allowing excessive suffering, but also do not avoid your feelings. Find a balance in this work where you allow yourself to feel the emotions you have been suppressing, while also remaining functional and enjoying the good life that Jesus died for you to have. We heal at the pace of grace.

Beloved, be sure to share your timeline work with at least one friend and pray frequently over this journey.

Take time now to go to your *Heart Journey*™ *Journal* and complete the **Individual Heartwork - Narrate Your Story**™ and the **Heart Group Discussion - Time to Share**.

## PRESSING ON

Moving forward, we have acquired RESOURCE™ skills and have started to uncover our stories. I commend you for your courage in facing your timelines, recognizing unmet needs and traumas, identifying recurring themes in your life, and embracing truth. This has been a lot to process. Take your time with this, Beloved. This *Heart Journey*™ has no time limits or pressures. Know you are loved and in God's hands. Cocoon into His support.

At this point, if your timeline looks like a jumble of a mess, do not worry, we will be able to use it as is. Can you feel hope and restoration knocking on the door of your heart? God is already working in the deep inner places. As Dory, in *Finding Nemo*, says, "Just keep swimming." And remember, He is with you, and He already paid the price for your healing. We are just learning how to receive all His goodness!

> *You've gone into my future to prepare the way, and in kindness You follow behind me to spare me from the harm of my past.*

Psalm 139:5 (TPT)

## LET US PRAY.

*Heavenly Father,*

*We thank You so much for our pasts … although they may not be pretty, we know you never waste a hurt. You will use it all!*

*Also, You specialize in turning ashes into beauty. Thank You, Father for taking our pasts and using them to make our futures bright. We love the fact that we do not have to settle for the enemy's agenda against our lives. Rather, we can embrace Your agenda for our lives and allow You to rewrite the narrative.*

*Thank You for being with us on this journey, Father. Help us to embrace all You have in store for us with open minds and hearts.*

*In Jesus' name, Amen.*

# Chapter

## SIX

### Restoring My Emotions

*Come to me, all you who are weary and burdened,*
*and I will give you rest.*
### Matthew 11:28 (NIV)

Have you ever felt driven into certain behaviors, relationships, or patterns, only to realize you are repeating a painful cycle again? Or have your ever experienced an underlying anxiety seeping into your relationships instead of the poise and confidence you desire. Oftentimes, when we had unmet needs as children, unsettled feelings and patterns can take hold of us, making it difficult to step into our fullness as a self-assured daughter of the King.

In this chapter, we delve into the "S" for Satisfy Unmet Needs™ in our RECONSTRUCTION™ acronym. We all have needs for belonging, connection, acceptance, safety, healthy boundaries, and validation, all of which translate into a secure home base from which to explore the world. If we did not have these needs met consistently, we function from an insecure base, which often sours our confidence and erodes our relationships with others, ourselves, and even God.

In this chapter, we will use encounters with Jesus, drawing, prayer, writing, somatic tools, and our holy imagination to finally give our souls the belonging, love, acceptance, and secure base for which we have longed.

## SATISFYING UNMET NEEDS™

*And my God will meet all your needs according to the riches of His glory in Christ Jesus.*

**Philippians 4:19 (NIV)**

Just like this Scripture states, God promises to meet our needs. But as children, most times we have no reason or knowledge to suspect our needs have been neglected. Yet as we enter into adulthood, we can scrutinize painful life and relationship cycles to find that our unmet needs from childhood are often the roots of these patterns.

As we continue reconstructing your heart home, our aim is to address your unmet needs, restore your emotions, and renovate the rooms of your heart home. Our goal is to help you fill the void of needs that were unmet in childhood and provide you with all that is good. Though unmet needs can be upsetting, Jesus is always available to meet every need with His love and grace. His Word is the source of the truth and wisdom we need to rebuild our heart homes.

Meeting our unmet needs creates a sense of wholeness and completeness rooted in God's love and value for us. We can trust God will provide for us, whether we need safety, security, love, or self-respect. As we continue on this *Heart Journey*™, we will explore different strategies and techniques for identifying and addressing our unmet needs, seeking the Lord's guidance and wisdom to lead us toward healing and wholeness.

To begin, we will examine Scriptures that reflect God's heart toward healing.

Psalm 27:1 (NIV) assures us that the Lord makes up for what was not there in our childhoods: Though my father and mother forsake me, The Lord will receive me.

Psalm 103:5 (NIV) reminds us that He wants to meet us at every age and stage of our lives: ... who satisfies your desires with good things so that your youth is renewed like the eagle's.

Joel 2:25-27 (NIV) promises that He will compensate us for the years that have been lost:

I will repay you for the years the locusts have eaten ... You will have plenty to eat, until you are full, and you will praise the name of the Lord your God, who has worked wonders for you; never again will my people be shamed. Then you will know that I am in Israel, that I am the Lord your God, and that there is no other ....

Using the tools in this chapter, we can experience God doing greater than we could ask or imagine, meeting us at each age and stage of our lives, adopting us as His children, as we move back through time via memory work. By addressing these unmet needs and themes, we can repair and strengthen our heart home, paving the way for success and joy in all aspects of our lives.

*Now to Him who is able to do immeasurably more than all we ask or imagine, according to His power that is at work within us.*

### Ephesians 3:20 (NIV)

Remember, Psalm 34:18 says, "The Lord is close to the brokenhearted and saves those who are crushed in spirit." Through our holy imagination, we can trust that God is present and able to heal our wounds, meeting our needs for belonging, nurture, security, safety, and protection.

## WHY SATISFY UNMET NEEDS?™

As you progressed through the narrative of your story in the last chapter, you identified specific and thematic unmet needs. Why is it important for us to work on these needs? Imagine that you enter your home and detect an unfamiliar and unpleasant odor. You attempt to discern its source by inspecting the refrigerator. Eventually, you discover a rotten onion, and you have to labor vigorously to eliminate the stench. You sanitize until your home smells pleasant once more. As long as you leave that onion there, however, the odor will persist and impact the atmosphere of your dwelling.

Likewise, our hearts are like homes that require the removal of toxic agents, which are akin to cancerous growths within us. These agents may manifest themselves via sabotaging our relationships, careers, callings, motherhood, or any aspect of our connections with others. It is difficult to achieve success with these elements seeping through the surface and infiltrating every nook and cranny of our lives.

As we reviewed earlier, our Scriptures affirm that the Lord desires to meet our unmet needs. When we envision God's presence without any restrictions, He is more than capable of healing our past wounds.

## ATTACHMENT: A DEEPER LOOK

As we noted earlier, we have certain needs as children that must be met for us to form secure attachments. Our attachment styles are shaped by early experiences with caregivers, and if those experiences were positive and nurturing, we are more likely to develop secure attachment. Secure attachment is an internal relational-emotional framework where we feel comfortable depending on others and have a sense of ourselves in relationships. It allows us to trust both ourselves and others in healthy ways and results in healthy connections with others. However, if we did not have our needs met in a proper manner, we may end up with insecure attachment styles.

As we discuss the four attachment types, consider reflecting on your own relationship history and identify which attachment style(s) resonates with you. This self-awareness can help you understand how past experiences with caregivers may have influenced your attachment style and how it may be affecting your current relationships. Then we will use our Satisfy Unmet Needs Tools™ to heal your attachment system.

There are four main types of attachment styles, and they are all tied back to our childhood needs. The first attachment style is secure attachment, where we feel comfortable depending on others and have a sense of ourselves in relationships. Our internal relational-emotional framework trusts both the self and others in a healthy manner. Secure attachment results from consistent and responsive caregiving. For instance, a child with secure attachment had their emotional and physical needs met by a parental caregiver, who was available and responsive to their needs. As adults, those with secure attachment tend to form healthy bonds at a healthy pace and have an inner sense of security within themselves, as well as a sense of security in their relationships.

The second attachment style is anxious attachment, also known as insecure-ambivalent attachment. People with this attachment style are often anxious and fearful of rejection, which can lead them to cling to others for security. They may lack trust in themselves and rely heavily on others to meet their needs. Women with anxious attachment may feel empty, like few others are truly there for them, even as they desperately reach out for connection. This attachment style can develop when caregivers are inconsistently available, and a child learns to cling to them when love is offered. For example, a child with this attachment style might have a caregiver who is not always present, leading the child to anxiously cling to them when they are available.

As adults, those with anxious attachment may quickly become emotionally invested in close relationships and have a strong belief that their needs can only be met by others. Additionally, they may struggle to fully accept the nourishment that others offer due to feeling it is not quite enough. Often, those with anxious attachment seek validation and intimacy in relationships, and tend to partner with those who avoid emotional closeness, prefer independence, and have avoidant attachment.

The third style is avoidant attachment style, also known as avoidant-dismissive attachment, and is characterized by a strong reluctance to engage in close relationships and a lack of trust in others. Individuals with this attachment style often fear emotional intimacy and believe it is only safe to rely on themselves. While they may feel a sense of loneliness, they prefer independence to the vulnerability and discomfort of emotional closeness. At times, people with avoidant attachment may enjoy the early stages of a relationship, but they may retreat when it comes to deeper intimacy and commitment. This attachment style typically develops when a caregiver is emotionally unavailable or unresponsive to a child's needs, causing the child to learn to avoid seeking emotional support in the future. The fear of being hurt again feels too frightening. As adults, although they may still desire connection, their fear of emotional closeness and vulnerability may be greater than their longing for connection.

The fourth type of attachment is disorganized attachment, which develops when a child experiences chaotic and confusing interactions with their caregiver, leading to difficulties in regulating their emotions and behaviors. Adults who grew up with parents with addictions may also develop this attachment style. Disorganized attachment often combines traits of both avoidant and anxious attachment styles. This attachment style typically arises in situations of abuse, neglect, or trauma. For instance, a child with disorganized attachment might have a caregiver who is abusive, resulting in confusion and an inability to regulate their emotions and behaviors. As adults, those with disorganized attachment may struggle to maintain healthy relationships, experiencing fight, flight, or freeze responses, especially when triggered. Individuals with disorganized attachment often feel they cannot trust themselves or others, leaving them with a deep longing for connection while also fearing it.

Beloved, as noted above, these attachment styles do not just affect childhood, but also manifest in adulthood. The good news is these attachment styles are not set in stone and can be changed. One powerful tool for healing unmet childhood needs is an encounter with Jesus within memory work. Let us recall that the Bible tells us that Jesus came to heal the brokenhearted and bind up our wounds (Psalm 147:3).

> *The Lord builds up Jerusalem; He gathers the exiles of Israel. He heals the brokenhearted and binds up their wounds.*
>
> ### Psalm 147:2-3 (NIV)

By turning to Him and welcoming Him to work within our greatest areas of need, we can experience profound healing and restoration. Additionally, our Satisfy Unmet Needs™ tools will draw us into more attachment system healing.

## MEMORY RECONSOLIDATION: A DEEPER LOOK

Our approach to healing and growth will involve a powerful combination of supernatural encounters with Jesus and cutting-edge scientific techniques that use a mechanism of change we highlighted in a previous chapter, called Memory Reconsolidation (MR).[21] Scientists believe that unlocking this mechanism involves the recollection and examination of memories, followed by introducing a "prediction error" within a specific time window of less than five hours.

When we work with negative memories, our brain expects negative consequences. In the *Heart Journey*™ Method, we will engage techniques that positively meet your childhood unmet needs as the "prediction error." For example, you will encounter Jesus and use Self-Momming™ to meet your childhood needs in memory work.

By engaging in carefully curated activities, we will create a safe and supportive space for your brain to reconsolidate old memories and form new, positive connections. Our goal is to help you overcome the effects of past experiences that may have left you feeling insecure and unloved, and to establish a secure and accepting foundation where your soul can flourish. This powerful combination of techniques will create the conditions for you to experience the transformative healing and internal sense of belonging for which you have been yearning.

## JESUS: THE ULTIMATE PREDICTION ERROR

In revisiting John 4:5-30, we can explore the powerful encounter Jesus had with a Samaritan woman at a well. As noted previously in our study, this woman was an outcast in her society due to her ethnicity and past experiences of divorce. Although we cannot limit Jesus' actions to a specific methodology, it is interesting to note how His approach aligned with the steps of Memory Reconsolidation (MR).

First, Jesus opened up the memories of her past by revealing her relationship history. Jesus revealed painful details about her five previous marriages and her current relationship status. However, He delivered this information gently and compassionately, creating a safe space for her to confront her past and form new, healthier connections in her brain.

Then, He demonstrated compassion and respect, engaging her in conversation and revealing Himself as the Messiah, her personal Savior. Her experience of His lavish love, juxtaposed to her felt humiliation, rejection, and shame, was likely the "prediction error" that changed her emotional learning.

By the end of their conversation, the woman's whole identity and countenance had been transformed from outcast to belonging. She went from hiding from others as an outcast to running toward others as a witness and evangelist for Jesus. She immediately proclaimed to her entire town the transformative power of His love and grace. This kind of profound change is precisely what Memory Reconsolidation aims to achieve. When we invite Jesus into our painful past, His love, truth, and belonging work together as a "prediction error" that causes emotional learning to change. By opening up old memories and introducing new, positive experiences with Jesus, the brain can form new neural connections that fundamentally make whole our internal world.

## SATISFY UNMET NEEDS™ TOOLS

We will work on Satisfying Unmet Needs™ in five ways: Quadruple Entry Journaling™, Oscillation, Pain to Purpose Drawing™, Restored Childhood with Jesus, and Empty Chair-Christian Version. All of these tools will work within the Memory Reconsolidation window and use encounters with Jesus.

## UNMET NEEDS

In the previous chapter, we discussed the vital developmental needs we had as children to become emotionally healthy and well-adjusted adult women. These needs included basic requirements such as safety, shelter, nourishment, clean water, and protection, as well as emotional needs such as secure attachment, a secure base, autonomy, emotional safety, validation, and boundaries.

Having these needs met was essential for us to develop healthy self-awareness, empathy, resilience to stress, problem-solving skills, and interpersonal skills. On the other hand, a lack of emotional safety, insecure attachment, and poor boundaries has led to emotional instability, poor emotional regulation, and anxiety for many of us. However, we can find comfort in knowing Jesus is here to restore what was lost.

Now it is time to reopen your *Heart Journey™ Journal* and complete the exercise in Chapter Six, **Individual Heartwork - Ordering Unmet Needs Memories.** You will work with your list of unmet needs from childhood and order the unmet needs and corresponding memories from least painful to most painful. We will use this list as we continue our Satisfy Unmet Needs™ Work.

Complete **Individual Heartwork - Ordering Unmet Needs Memories** within your *Heart Journey™ Journal* at this time.

Beloved, great work! We will use this list later in this chapter. We will titrate our work, which means we will work with the least painful memories first, and work our way into the most painful. And remember, use your RESOURCE™ skills frequently to regulate your emotions and nervous system.

## PARTS WORK

Have you ever experienced the joy of opening a Russian nesting doll with the excitement of discovering each smaller doll within the larger one? In the same way, I believe each of us has parts of ourselves that make up our internal relational-emotional world.

The concept of Parts Work in inner healing suggests that our internal world is composed of various mental states associated with unique emotions, memories, beliefs, and behaviors. When certain triggers are encountered, these parts can be activated, resulting in a state—dependent memory effect. This means we are more likely to remember events when our current emotional and physiological state matches the state we were in when we first encoded the memory.

In the context of Christian inner healing, our ultimate objective is to integrate these distinct parts of ourselves with Jesus to foster a whole and Christ-filled response to triggers in the future. In working with these parts of ourselves, we constantly take them to Jesus.

Our parts of self can be both adult-like and childlike. For instance, your adult parts may urge you to eat broccoli, while your child parts may crave pie. Healthy child parts are playful, but burdened and unhealed child parts tend to express in one of three variations when we are triggered: the highly vulnerable and wounded child, the child that acts out, and the overbearing inner critic.

Usually, the wounded part of us is hidden beneath the critical and acting-out parts that serve as defense mechanisms to keep the wounded parts concealed. It is normative to experience parts of ourselves and not pathological. Have you ever said, "Part of me wants to ... ?" God wants every part of us to be healed and saturated with Jesus.

Research has shown that traumatic experiences can lead to changes in the brain's neural networks, which can result in wound-based patterns of thinking, feeling, and behavior. Parts Work seeks to address these wound-based patterns by helping to identify and work with the specific parts of the psyche associated with these patterns. Many therapy modalities use Parts Work including Richard Schwartz's Internal Family Systems and Jeffery Young's Schema Therapy.[22]

Here is an example of how a child part might become wounded and express herself throughout life. Jessie experiences social anxiety, especially when in group get-togethers. A part of herself is always on the lookout for danger when in a group of peers. This part may be a child part stuck in fourth grade, when Jessie was bullied by a group of girls for the entire year. By identifying and allowing Jesus to work with this part, Jessie can reprogram the neural pathways linked to social anxiety.

Jesus wants to heal, comfort, and unburden our parts of self. Let us reflect on Psalm 23 (TPT) in The Passion Translation to hear His heart for our vulnerable parts of self.

Yahweh is my best friend and my shepherd.
I always have more than enough.
He offers a resting place for me in His luxurious love.
His tracks take me to an oasis of peace
near the quiet brook of bliss.
That's where He restores and revives my life.
He opens before me the right path
and leads me along in His footsteps of righteousness
so that I can bring honor to His name.
Even when Your path takes me through
the valley of deepest darkness,
fear will never conquer me, for You already have!
Your authority is my strength and my peace.
The comfort of Your love takes away my fear.
I'll never be lonely, for You are near.
You become my delicious feast
even when my enemies dare to fight.
You anoint me with the fragrance of Your Holy Spirit;
You give me all I can drink of You until my cup overflows.
So why would I fear the future?
Only goodness and tender love pursue me all the days of my life.
Then afterward, when my life is through,
I'll return to Your glorious presence to be forever with You!

Beloved, Parts Work can be understood as a way to amalgamate our inner selves with God's love and person. By exploring and allowing Him to heal our wounded child parts, we become more whole and integrated with Him. This aligns with the biblical concept of sanctification, which is the process of becoming more like Christ (Romans 8:29). As we heal and integrate different parts of ourselves, we can become more aligned with God's will and better equipped to fulfill our radiant God-ordained purpose in life.

*For those whom He foreknew [and loved and chose beforehand], He also predestined to be conformed to the image of His Son [and ultimately share in His complete sanctification], so that He would be the firstborn [the most beloved and honored] among many believers.*

### Romans 8:29 (AMP)

One of my favorite Bible stories regarding the restoration of vulnerable parts of self is the story of Mephibosheth in 2 Samuel Chapter 9. Saul and Jonathan had been killed in war with the Philistines, and David had been installed as king of Israel.

After King David established his Kingdom, he remembered his brotherly love for Saul's son, Jonathan, and asked his attendants if there was anyone left from Saul's house that he could bless for Jonathan's sake. King David went down to a place called LoDebar and found Jonathan's son, Mephibosheth, who had been dropped by his nursemaid while fleeing town when his father, Jonathan, was killed. She fled with Mephibosheth out of fear that the rest of Saul's house would be killed with the shifting of kingdoms.

When David arrived at LoDebar, he called out, "Mephibospeth." Mephibosheth came out of hiding and fell on his face, saying, "What would you do with a dead dog like me?" Interestingly, Mephibosheth, Saul's heir, had full rights to establish himself as a king, but instead, he saw himself so lowly that he compared himself to a dead dog.

In kindness, David restored all the kingdoms of Saul to Mephibosheth. The Scripture then says that Mephibosheth ate at the king's table all the days of his life, "even though he was lame in both feet."

This story reminds me that God wants us to bring the most vulnerable parts of ourselves to His table every day. Similarly, Father God asks, "Who can I bless for Jesus' sake?" Just as David called out "Mephibosheth," God is calling out to your most vulnerable parts to fellowship with Him. He is saying, "Let the little children come to me." He seeks out the most vulnerable, shame-filled parts of our inner hearts to bring them out of hiding in LoDebar to a lavish feast of love and soul care. For this reason, dear one, we will give Him access to our child parts of self as we complete our Satisfy Unmet Needs work™.

Additionally, Paul provides a powerful analogy of the church as a body composed of many parts in 1 Corinthians 12:16-26. Each part is essential and plays a unique role, even those that may seem weaker or less honorable.

God has intentionally designed each part and bestowed greater honor on those that lacked it. This unity ensures no division within the body and that all members care for one another. By applying this analogy to our internal parts, we can see that God desires to bring honor to every part of us, even the more vulnerable ones. He wants to integrate all parts of us into wholeness, so we can function together in alignment with him.

## DEBORAH'S STORY

Let us return to our friend Deborah as an example. You likely recall that Deborah grew up with a mother who constantly rejected her and told her, "I hate you." At the age of thirteen, Deborah was emotionally devastated by her mother's words and felt like a small, helpless child desperate for love. Recently, Deborah experienced a similar emotional struggle when her boss criticized her work in front of colleagues. In that moment, she felt like a vulnerable and wounded child once again, even though she is an accomplished professional in her field. Deborah worked through her *Heart Journey*™ *Journal Heartwork*, and her Parts Work looked like this:

*The child that acts out: This part of Deborah is reactive and impulsive. When her boss criticized her work, this part of her wanted to lash out and defend herself, even if it meant being disrespectful, defensive, and critical. In addition, she went home and ate a container of fudge icing.*

*The overbearing inner critic: This part of Deborah is harsh and critical, and it often tells her that she is not good enough. In the moment of the criticism, this part of her said things like "No one likes you," "You're defective," and "Everyone thinks you're incompetent." These thoughts flooded her mind for several days after this incident.*

*The highly vulnerable and wounded child: This part of Deborah is deeply hurt by rejection and criticism. When her boss criticized her work, this part of her felt like a small and helpless child once again, and she was overwhelmed by sadness, fear, and shame. She felt unlovable and worthy of hate.*

We must bring healing to these child parts into the full life of the Spirit. In Romans 8:6 (NIV), Scripture says, "The mind governed by the flesh is death, but the mind governed by the Spirit is life and peace." This means that when we allow the wounds of our past to dictate our present responses, we are operating in the mind of the flesh. However, when we take these wounded parts of ourselves to Jesus for healing, we can experience the life and peace of the Spirit. By allowing the Holy Spirit to heal our wounded parts, we can experience the abundant life that Jesus promised in John 10:10 (ESV): "I came that they may have life and have it abundantly."

## SHAME

Dear friend, as we engage in the process of working with the different parts of ourselves and exploring memories related to unmet needs, the felt sense of shame will inevitably arise. Shame has been present since the beginning of humanity when Adam and Eve ran and hid from God and attempted to cover their disgrace.

According to Brené Brown, researcher on shame and vulnerability, shame is the intensely painful feeling or experience of believing we are flawed and therefore unworthy of love and belonging.[23] However, as Christians, we know Jesus paid the price for our shame and offers us a double portion of His grace and love.

As we continue to work with the inner parts of our heart, it takes great courage to face our shame. At the same time, it is important to understand that shame is an inherent part of the human experience.

The lie of shame is that we are uniquely defective, and therefore utterly unlovable. Rather, we are all victims of shame through the curse (Genesis 3; Deuteronomy 28; Romans 3:23), yet Jesus came to set us free from this tormenting shackle (Galatians 3:13). Jesus rose in power to set us free from shame and to offer us extravagant healing and restoration. We died and rose with Him when we believed in Him (Romans 6:4).

By embracing the profound power of the cross and resurrection, we have the incredible opportunity to bring our burdened souls to Jesus, inviting Him into every crevice tainted by the venomous grip of shame. In His boundless grace, He liberates us, enabling us to soar with newfound freedom, as His finished work on the cross washes away every stain, leaving us cleansed and renewed. Remember, it is our most vulnerable parts of self that feel the most shame, stuck in LoDebar, that He welcomes to sit and eat at His lavish table of love and soul care.

Now it is time to complete your **Individual Heartwork - Parts of Self** from your *Heart Journey*™ *Journal*. You will explore Parts of Self that are present in a current emotional struggle.

## QUADRUPLE ENTRY JOURNALING™ TOOL

Now that we have identified your personal unmet needs in your timeline work and discovered your own inner parts of self, we will use our Quadruple Entry Journaling™ tool to help you address them.

## PNEUMACEPTION™

Let us take a moment to explore the concept of Pneumaception™ before we delve into the practical application of Quadruple Entry Journaling™. This skill is rooted in the Greek word *"pneuma"*, life-giving vapor or Spirit, and the suffix *"ception,"* notice or sense. Pneumaception™ enables us to sense and perceive the presence and movement of the Holy Spirit, allowing us to be attuned to His leading and voice.

In John 10:27 (NKJV) Jesus said, "My sheep hear My voice, and I know them, and they follow Me." Clearly, Jesus said we can hear Him. Through Pneumaception™, we can encounter Jesus as He is always speaking to us through our spiritual senses.

Jesus also said He only does what He sees His father doing, and as children of God, we are also led by Him according to Romans 8:14 (NKJV), which states, "For as many as are led by the Spirit of God, these are sons of God." Therefore, He is always leading us and speaking to us.

By Pnuemacepting™, we tune into His frequency and can see, hear, sense, and feel what He is saying through our spiritual senses. This is similar to tuning into a radio frequency. The Scripture often speaks of seeing, hearing, and even tasting the Lord (Psalm 34:8; Hebrews 6:5). Hearing Him is a learned skill we improve with over time as we grow in intimacy with Him. In Quadruple Entry Journaling™, we will be tuning into the Holy Spirit and receiving the frequency of His voice.

*Oh, taste and see that the Lord is good;*
*Blessed is the man who trusts in Him!*

**Psalm 34:8 (NKJV)**

*...and have tasted the good word of God*
*and the powers of the age to come.*

**Hebrews 6:5 (NKJV)**

**Self-Momming**™. We will also be using our Self-Momming™ tool, which is one of our RESOURCE™ tools that allows us to meet our unmet childhood needs in the present day, using Jesus as our model parent. It involves nurturing and guiding ourselves, providing comfort and encouragement during times of struggle by the power of the Holy Spirit.

As a review, adults become our own parents and have to lead ourselves like parents would children. However, most of us have internalized a harsh inner critic rather than a nurturing, validating, and wise parent. The Self-Momming™ tool helps us replace this inner voice with an internal wise and nurturing parent governed by the love and wisdom of God. We achieve this by asking Jesus how He wants to parent us in a stressful situation, listening to His voice, and nurturing our inner child with His love and acceptance. It is essential to participate and agree with His nurturing by treating ourselves the same way.

**It's Over.** It is important to acknowledge that your past is over, and that you have survived it. You have the strength to seek healing and wisdom, and you have a personal and real relationship with the Lord, the ultimate healer.

As we work on addressing each unmet need, remember you always have yourself, God, and the resources available to you in adulthood, whether through your career, family, or community. You also have a powerful skill within you—your ability to Self-Mom™. So, continue to remind yourself that the past is over, and you are safe, as you engage in Memory Reconsolidation work.

**Memory Accuracy**. Perceptions can heavily influence our internal reality regarding beliefs and memories, and as Christians, we are aware of the enemy's ability to manipulate here. When it comes to memories, it is essential to acknowledge they are often colored by our perceptions, which may not always align with an objective reality.

As an example, research demonstrates that eyewitness reports can be unreliable due to the different perspectives people have.[24] In addition, memories can become less accurate over time.[25] Nonetheless, by focusing on the perception that has taken root within us, we can use the Satisfy Unmet Needs™ tools to have a restorative and healing experience. Therefore, we will be working with your perceptions of what you remember happening, while realizing our memories are corroded by time and perception.

## DEBORAH'S QUADRUPLE ENTRY JOURNALING™

To help get you started, here is Deborah's Quadruple Entry Journaling™ Work:

**Memory**. When Deborah was five-and-a-half years old, her brother was born. She felt a need for someone to explain what was happening and stay connected with her during that time.

**Unmet Needs.** Deborah experienced unmet needs for connection, compassion, healthy communication, acceptance, and emotional safety.

**Child Part Feelings.** Deborah experienced fear, anxiety, vulnerability, and abandonment. She felt scared and anxious due to the lack of connection and communication from her family members. She longed for someone to talk to her and make her feel safe and secure.

**Encounter with Jesus.** Deborah asked Jesus into this memory. He took her hand, paid special attention to her, explained everything, and treated her as His "little princess." She softened into this special love and nurture.

**Self-Momming™.** Deborah found it easier to receive Jesus' love than to Self-Mom™ her child parts. She reflected on how God made little Deborah and thought about her loveable niece, making progress with feeling and extending love toward her child parts. She spoke to her younger self as a mother in her memory, saying internally, "I love you sweet Deborah, and I am with you. You are special to me, and you will always be the most special girl in the world to me. As your brother comes home, I will not leave you. Jesus will not leave you. We are so close to you and will never leave you alone."

**Receiving from Safe Others.** Deborah added safe others to her memory, ensuring that every need was met. She brought in her paternal grandparents, who assured and nurtured her.

As Deborah finished working with this memory, she felt a new sense of comfort and belonging in her heart home.

*All your children shall be taught by the Lord*
*and great shall be the peace of your children.*

Isaiah 54:13 (NIV)

## IDEAL PARENTING BY STAGE

As you work on meeting your needs in your Quadruple Entry Journaling™, it may be helpful to understand how skillful, nurturing, protective, and guiding parents interact with their children at the different stages of life. Below are brief descriptions you can use as you practice Self-Momming™:

**Zero to Two Years.** Nurturing parents of infants focus on meeting their baby's needs for food, comfort, and safety, and are responsive to their cries for attention. They hold, cuddle, and soothe their little one with loving touch, reassuring words, and eye contact. Protective parents create a safe, predictable environment for their child to explore and learn in. Guiding parents model healthy routines, such as regular naps and bedtime, and provide age-appropriate toys and activities that stimulate their baby's senses. Spiritually nurturing parents introduce their child to God through simple prayers, blessings, and Bible stories, and model a life of faith and trust in God's love and care.

**Three to Five Years.** Nurturing parents of preschoolers continue to provide physical and emotional care and support, while also encouraging their child's growing independence and self-expression. They listen attentively to their child's questions, ideas, and stories, and engage in imaginative play and creative projects together. Protective parents set clear boundaries and rules, and help their child learn to manage their emotions and behaviors. Guiding parents offer opportunities for their child to explore the world around them, learn new skills, and develop a sense of curiosity and wonder. Spiritually nurturing parents help their child develop spiritual disciplines such as prayer, gratitude, and kindness, and encourage them to participate in simple acts of worship and service.

**Six to Ten Years.** Nurturing parents of elementary-age children provide emotional support and encouragement as their child navigates new social and academic challenges. They offer praise and constructive feedback, and help their child build confidence and resilience. Protective parents continue to set boundaries and monitor their child's activities and relationships, while also allowing for more autonomy and responsibility. Guiding parents encourage their child's curiosity and critical thinking, and provide opportunities for them to explore their interests and passions. Spiritually nurturing parents help their child develop a deeper understanding of God's love and plan for their life, and encourage them to develop habits of prayer, Bible reading, and serving others.

**Eleven to Fourteen Years.** Nurturing parents of pre-teens and early teens offer emotional support and guidance as their child faces the challenges of adolescence, including puberty, peer pressure, and academic stress. They maintain open communication and listen non-judgmentally to their child's concerns and struggles. Protective parents continue to set limits and provide structure, while also respecting their child's growing need for independence and privacy. Guiding parents help their child develop critical thinking skills and decision-making abilities, and provide opportunities for them to explore their identity and interests. Spiritually nurturing parents encourage their child to develop a personal relationship with God, and help them understand the relevance of faith to their everyday life.

**Fifteen to Eighteen Years.** Nurturing parents of teenagers offer emotional support and affirmation, while also helping their child prepare for adulthood and increased responsibility. They respect their child's growing autonomy, while also offering guidance and advice when needed. Protective parents continue to set limits and provide guidance, while also respecting their child's growing maturity and independence. Guiding parents encourage their child to develop a sense of purpose and direction, and help them explore career and educational opportunities. Spiritually nurturing parents help their child develop a mature and authentic faith, and encourage them to seek God's guidance and wisdom in all aspects of their life.

**Nineteen to Twenty-five Years.** Nurturing parents of young adults offer emotional support and encouragement, while also respecting their child's growing independence and adult responsibilities. They provide a safe and supportive home environment, while also allowing their child to pursue their own goals and dreams. Protective parents offer guidance and advice as needed, while also respecting their child's right to make their own decisions. Guiding parents of young adults help their children to develop spiritual disciplines and a strong faith foundation, while also encouraging them to explore and ask questions about their beliefs. They provide resources and guidance for their child to navigate the challenges of adulthood, including relationships, career, and personal growth.

**Twenty-five Years Onward.** Nurturing, protective, and guiding parents of adult children encourage independence and provide support as needed. They respect their children's autonomy and offer guidance and advice when asked. They continue to model healthy boundaries and communication, and they foster a relationship of mutual respect and trust. From a Christian perspective, they also continue to encourage spiritual growth and provide opportunities for their children to deepen their relationship with God and serve in their communities.

Overall, excellent parents who are nurturing, protective, and guiding strive to create an environment that fosters growth, independence, and healthy relationships with God and others. By practicing Self-Momming™ within your Quadruple Entry Journaling™ and learning from the brief descriptions provided for each age group, you can work toward meeting your own unmet needs with Jesus. You and Jesus can provide the nurturing, protective, and guiding presence your inner child needs. This can help you develop a healthier and more fulfilling relationship with yourself and with others, and also deepen your spiritual journey.

## INDIVIDUAL HEARTWORK – QUADRUPLE ENTRY JOURNALING™

Quadruple Entry Journaling™ is our main tool for meeting unmet needs. The other tools in this chapter will be utilized for those memories that still feel unresolved after this activity. You will work on each memory from your Ordering Unmet Needs Memories, one at a time, starting with your least painful memory.

Complete **Individual Heartwork - Quadruple Entry Journaling™** within your *Heart Journey™ Journal* at this time.

After working through your memories using Quadruple Entry Journaling™, it is time to inspect for things from the past that still seem to ache in your heart.

## STICKY MEMORIES

In your *Heart Journey™ Journal*, you will make a list of the memories that still feel stuck. In other words, you will explore your work, and look for Unmet Needs memories where you were not able to access a felt sense of your needs being met. We will learn several tools to work with these Sticky Memories.

Complete **Individual Heartwork - Sticky Unmet Needs Memories™** within your *Heart Journey™ Journal* at this time.

## WORKING WITH STICKY MEMORIES

Next, we will learn several tools for working with Sticky Memories, all of which use traditions of our faith as well as Memory Reconsolidation underpinnings. We will learn Oscillation with Jesus™, Pain to Purpose Drawing™, and Empty Chair-Christian Version.

## OSCILLATION WITH JESUS™

One of the tools we use with Sticky Memories is "Oscillation with Jesus™." You might recall that the Oscillation tool is used to process and resolve Unmet Needs or Trauma Triggers by following an imaginary figure-eight with a positive and negative stimulus associated with the trauma. The technique involves opening up the trauma memory with the negative stimulus and simultaneously creating a "prediction error" with the positive stimulus. By oscillating back and forth between the positive and negative stimuli, we can facilitate the integration of new, positive emotional learning into the memory and reduce the emotional distress associated with it.

Complete **Individual Heartwork - Oscillation with Jesus**™ within your *Heart Journey*™ *Journal* at this time.

Use this QR code to access audible versions of activities.

## PAIN TO PURPOSE DRAWING™

The next tool we will use on Sticky Memories is "Pain to Purpose Drawing™." You will need colored pencils or markers for this activity. Here, we will draw a set of three pictures for each Sticky Memory™ with which you want to use this tool.

Complete **Individual Heartwork - Pain to Purpose Drawing**™ within your *Heart Journey*™ *Journal* at this time.

## BEAUTIFUL PLACE PRAYER™

As children of God, we know our pain and traumas are not the end of the story. The Lord has promised to take our brokenness and turn it into something beautiful, as we see in the lives of many characters in the Bible.

For example, let us recall again Joseph's brothers sold him into slavery, but God used that situation to elevate him to a position of power in Egypt, where he was able to save his family from famine (Genesis 50:20). Similarly, Job suffered immense loss and pain, but through his trials, he gained a deeper understanding of God's sovereignty and was blessed with even greater abundance (Job 42:10-17).

One powerful tool for dealing with our pain is to commit it to the Lord and ask Him to turn it into something beautiful. This is called the Beautiful Place Prayer™. We can trust that God is faithful and that He will work all things together for good for those who love Him (Romans 8:28). By surrendering our pain to Him, letting go of all bitterness, and inviting Him to turn it into a Beautiful Place, we set in motion His healing and restoration in our lives. If we ask for the bread of healing, He will not give us a stone (Matthew 7:9-11).

## DEBORAH'S STORY

Our friend Deborah's experience of loss and pain led her to pray the Beautiful Place Prayer™. As she surrendered her pain to the Lord and asked Him to show her how He could turn it into something beautiful, God began to heal her heart and bring her fulfillment through ministry work.

One of the areas where Deborah found herself ministering most effectively was on the topic of child loss. Her personal experience of a full-term stillbirth gave her a unique perspective and empathy for others who have gone through similar experiences. By doing her own Heartwork and trusting God through the Beautiful Place Prayer™, Deborah was able to find healing and restoration, and use her story to bring hope and comfort to others who were hurting.

Through her ministry work, Deborah was able to see God take her pain and turn it into something beautiful. She became like a spiritual mother to many, and the love and care she poured into the lives of others brought her great joy and fulfillment. Deborah's life is a testament to the power of surrendering our pain to God and trusting Him to turn it into something beautiful.

Complete **Individual Heartwork - Beautiful Place Prayer**™ within your *Heart Journey*™ *Journal* at this time.

## EMPTY CHAIR-CHRISTIAN VERSION

The "Empty Chair-Christian Version" is a powerful tool that can help you work with Sticky Memories that involve a situation with another where you did not feel you had a voice. The "Empty Chair-Christian Version" involves imagining the person sitting in an empty chair across from you, then using your voice to express how their actions affected you. This technique can help you heal old wounds, release pent-up emotions, and move forward with greater clarity and peace.

Complete **Individual Heartwork - Empty Chair-Christian Version** within your *Heart Journey*™ *Journal* at this time.

Use this QR code to access audible versions of activities.

## RESTORED CHILDHOOD WITH JESUS

The Restored Childhood with Jesus Activity is a transformative tool that utilizes your holy imagination to help you encounter Jesus. He will meet the unmet needs from your childhood as you allow Jesus to restore and fill the gaps of your childhood experiences.

Complete **Individual Heartwork - Restored Childhood with Jesus Activity** within your *Heart Journey*™ *Journal* at this time.

Use this QR code to access audible versions of activities.

Wow, we have really Satisfied Unmet Needs™, Beloved! As we close out this chapter and prepare to move into Time Reversing Trauma™, let us take some time to explore grief.

## CHILDHOOD LOSSES AND UNCOVERED GRIEF

Working through childhood memories, losses, and traumas can be a difficult and emotional process. Christians (and other religious women and men) can combine the skills and tools of faith and psychology to navigate through it successfully. One essential tool is to trust in

God's comfort and love during times of grief. One of our keystone scriptures states, "The LORD is close to the brokenhearted and saves those who are crushed in spirit" (Psalm 34:18 NIV). By placing our trust in God's promise to be with us during difficult times, we can find comfort and hope.

In addition to seeking comfort in our faith, it is also important to allow ourselves time to process our grief feelings. By scheduling time to work through our sorrow, we can better manage unexpected "grief attacks" and find a healthier, happier balance in our lives. While working through our grief, self-compassion is key. Practicing self-compassion can be achieved through Self-Momming™, which reminds us it is okay to feel sad and that we are worthy of love and care.

Another helpful tool for working through grief is writing letters to our child parts after doing inner child work through Quadruple Entry Journaling™. Writing letters to our inner child can help us process emotions and provide comfort to the hurting parts of ourselves. We can acknowledge the pain and losses our child parts experienced while offering words of affirmation, comfort, and hope. This can help us heal from past traumas and losses, and move forward with a greater sense of wholeness and self-love.

It is important to remember that healing from childhood losses and working through grief is a journey that takes time. It is okay to take things at our own pace and seek out support from trusted friends, family, or licensed mental health professionals if needed. By using a combination of faith and psychological skills, we can navigate through the process of healing and find a sense of peace and wholeness.

Complete **Individual Heartwork - Childhood Losses and Uncovered Grief** within your *Heart Journey™ Journal* at this time.

I am thrilled with all you are accomplishing, Beloved. Be sure to finish your **Individual Heartwork - Chapter Six Review** and your **Heart Group Discussion** work with your small group or with a friend. In the next chapter, we continue to rebuild your heart as we Time Reverse Traumas™.

## LET US PRAY.

*Heavenly Father,*

*We come before You with grateful hearts, asking for Your healing touch upon our hearts and memories. Lord, we pray that You would go into every nook and cranny of our heart homes, removing everything the enemy intended for evil and replacing it with Your love, acceptance, belonging, wholeness, and healing. We pray for freedom from the chains that bind us and speak freedom in the mighty name of Jesus.*

*Holy Spirit, we invite You into this place, blessing and making Yourself at home. We ask that You renovate and reconstruct our hearts and memories, pouring out Your Spirit upon us. Lord, we pray that there would be no space left unturned or unhealed in our memories. Meet every need, Lord, and heal every space in our hearts.*

*Father, we thank You that right now, hearts are being healed and receiving You in new ways. We welcome You into every room, every corner, and every storage space of our hearts. We pray that there would be no distance between us and You in any space. Thank You for seeking out every lost place within us, like the woman who had nine coins but looked for the one lost one.*

*Lord, we thank You that every part of ourselves comes to the table, just like Mephibosheth ate at the king's table. We thank You for continuing this healing work and for adopting each part of each person to Yourself, joining them to their forever home in You.*

*In Jesus' name, Amen.*

# Chapter

## SEVEN

### Restoring My Security

*You will keep in perfect and constant peace the one whose mind is
steadfast [that is, committed and focused on You—in both inclination
and character], Because He trusts and takes refuge in You [with hope
and confident expectation].*

### Isaiah 26:3 (AMP)

Restoring peace through reversing the impact of trauma will
ignite a major shift in the atmosphere of our renovated heart
homes. In this chapter, we continue working through our acronym,
and the "T" in RECONSTRUCTION™ stands for "Time Reverse
Trauma™." The techniques we will use will help us to break free from
places where we have been stuck in the past, but we will do so at a
pace that is manageable. Through this measure of our journey, we will
deepen our understanding of trauma, renegotiating its impact section
by section, while harmonizing and regulating our nervous system
through encounters with Jesus. Additionally, we will compassionately

address the body's innate responses, such as orienting, defending, and the fight-or-flight instinct, ultimately finding resolution that ushers in an abundance of God's joy, tranquility, and solace.

## ORDERING TRAUMAS

To begin, we will look at your list of traumas from Chapter Five and order them from least to most painful. We will titrate by working on the least painful first. Recollect that with trauma work, slow is fast. As we metabolize the lesser traumas, it is easier to metabolize those that are greater.

Complete **Individual Heartwork - Ordering Traumas** within your *Heart Journey*™ *Journal* at this time.

## TIME REVERSE TRAUMA™ OVERVIEW

We will be utilizing the powerful *Heart Journey*™ method of Time Reverse Trauma™, which is designed to unlock Memory Reconciliation and emotional healing. Our approach will involve carefully and gently working through each traumatic memory, one slice at a time, starting at the edges (T-7 and T+7) and gradually moving toward the heart of the trauma (T=0). By dividing the trauma into manageable slices, we will be able to process it more effectively.

Throughout this chapter, we will use various techniques to help us process and heal. We will spend time writing or drawing about what happened, and we will identify the resources we needed in that memory. We will also identify any orienting, flight, or fight responses that needed to be completed, and we will use our holy imagination to invite Jesus in to give us what we needed at each slice of the trauma situation. We will also allow ourselves to have every resource we need and allow for every nervous system response to be completed, while holding the hand of Jesus every step of the way.

Once we have used the Time Reverse Trauma™ method to work through our traumas, we will then explore our Sticky Memories. In these hard-to-resolve traumas, we will use Oscillation with Jesus™ and Pain to Purpose Drawing™ to help us find resolution and healing. Finally, we will conclude our work with the Beautiful Place Prayer™, bringing closure and peace to our hearts.

## RESOURCE™ OUR WAY THROUGH

This chapter may be particularly challenging, so before we jump in, let us take a moment to ground ourselves and review some tools that we can use to prevent overwhelm. One set of skills that we can draw from is the RESOURCE™ model, which includes twenty-five different techniques to help build stability and resilience in the face of difficult experiences. These skills include reframing our thoughts through techniques like Inventorying Your Thinking or Mind Mansion™, enriching our lives with positive memories and Safe Place imagery, and Undergirding with Support with safe people. We can also use relaxation skills like Christian Progressive Relaxation or 5, 4, 3, 2, 1 Meditation-Christian Version to help calm our nervous system and Occupy Our Body through Grounding and Tracking techniques.

Additionally, we can work on Structuring Our Lives through self-care, life editing, and practicing different types of rest. Finally, we can use techniques like Oscillation and Titration to gradually work through difficult experiences and move toward acceptance and change. By drawing on these skills, we can support ourselves as we work through the challenging material in this chapter. Remember to use your RESOURCE™ skills and move at the pace of grace so that you remain within the Window of Tolerance.

## DISTANCING STRATEGIES

In this chapter, it will be important to remember to use our Distancing Strategies to regulate our nervous system when memory content becomes overwhelming. Our first strategy, Binoculars Backwards™, involves mentally zooming out from the painful memory to create distance. The second strategy is the Movie Screen Strategy, where we visualize the memory content on an external screen. Lastly, the "It's Over" Strategy reminds us that the painful event has concluded, and we are safe now. To stay within the Window of Tolerance and avoid dissociation, it is vital to recall the relief we felt when the event ended and repeat the affirmation, "It's over. I survived, and God is going to turn my ashes into beauty."

## DEALING WITH OVERWHELM

If the techniques discussed in this chapter evoke strong emotions that push you to the edge of your Window of Tolerance, it is important to remember your resources. To cope with overwhelming emotions, it is crucial to keep the experience manageable by relying on our support system, moving at the pace of grace, and using your RESOURCE™ tools. You can confide in your small group facilitator, your prayer/accountability partner, or a licensed psychotherapist you trust. If you ever feel unsafe, it is important to put the work down and call 911 immediately.

In summary, addressing trauma is challenging, but it is important to move forward where you can, manageably. With the help of our support system, reliance on our RESOURCE™ skills, putting safety first, and focusing on Jesus, we can get through overwhelming experiences and improve our well-being.

## COMPLETING INCOMPLETE TRAUMA RESPONSES

When we experience traumatic events, our natural nervous system process may be interrupted, preventing us from completing the instinctive reactions such as fight or flight. For instance, if we are attacked, we may feel the urge to fight back or run away, but we may be unable to do so. As we heal, we can use our holy imagination to complete these incomplete responses and integrate the traumatic experiences properly into our nervous system.

Somatic therapies emphasize the importance of completing these instinctive responses as a fundamental aspect of healing. By engaging in this process, we allow our nervous system to fully process and integrate the trauma, involving areas such as the hippocampus, prefrontal cortex, and amygdala. For instance, in the context of a car accident, the rapid occurrence of the event may have prevented us from fully orienting ourselves and utilizing defensive reactions. Fulfilling the incomplete responses can involve using our holy imagination to envision ourselves responding in a way that we were unable to at that moment, facilitating the healing and integration of the traumatic experience within our nervous system to completion.

In other cases, such as sexual assault, completing the response might involve imagining fighting back or escaping the attacker's grasp. This process of using our holy imagination to complete unfinished responses can be powerful in healing trauma and integrating it into our nervous system. It allows us to reclaim a sense of agency and control over our experiences, which can be empowering and transformative.

## FROM ALONE TO CONNECTION

When you process your trauma memories, it is imperative to reimagine each slice of the memory with safe support so that we do not feel alone during the process. You can insert a variety of safe attachment figures, including safe people and Jesus, to accompany you before, during, and after each memory portion. As you revisit the trauma, you can also rework and reimagine elements of the memory to meet the unmet needs in the memory. For example, if you were alone during a traumatic event, you can add comforting others and spiritual support from the Godhead to the memory. You can also bring in Self as Mom™. This can help you establish a sense of security and comfort, and facilitate our healing from the trauma.

Complete **Individual Heartwork - From Alone to Connection** within your *Heart Journey™ Journal* at this time.

## APPROACHING TRAUMATIC MEMORIES WITH CARE

Memory can be a difficult and unreliable aspect of trauma, especially as memories are processed differently during traumatic events so encoding can be partial or skewed. Therefore, if there is uncertainty about the validity of a traumatic memory, it is not advisable to push for more details, but rather, work with the available information and move on. The process is similar to that of Satisfy Unmet Needs™, where we focus on our perception of what happened, while acknowledging that memory is flawed and limited in scope.

It is important to approach the possibility of false memories with precaution, as they can be more damaging than helpful. We avoid engaging in suggestive narratives where details are lacking. To avoid this, we can take a gentle approach and focus on the sensory details and emotions that we remember.

Additionally, we can acknowledge the natural limitations of memory and remain open-minded and flexible in our perceptions and interpretations of our experiences. This will help us to work with what we remember while trusting the Lord to guide us through the unknowns. By being watchful, cautious, and accepting of the limitations of memory, we can work toward a balanced understanding of our experiences.

## MEETING NEEDS WITHIN TRAUMAS

In your Time Reversing Trauma™ Heartwork, we will approach Memory Reconsolidation with the same goal as in our work with Satisfying Unmet Needs™: to meet the needs that were not met during the traumatic event. We have already noted that many scientists believe that Memory Reconsolidation is a process by which emotional learning within a memory is modified and updated with new information, and to achieve this, we first open up the memory by recalling the emotions, body sensations, and details from the recollection. Then, within five hours of opening the memory, we create a prediction error by introducing a positive stimulus that meets the needs that were unmet during the traumatic event. This is important because the brain is not expecting needs to be met, but rather anticipates something awful to happen, so meeting those needs can help to create a sense of safety and healing.

A traumatic experience can shatter our sense of safety and leave us with a variety of needs that must be addressed during the healing and reconciliation process. Some of these needs might include:

1.  Safety: During the traumatic event, we may have felt a sense of danger, vulnerability, and fear, and our need for safety and security became paramount. We had to find ways to protect ourselves and establish a sense of safety.

2.  Connection: Trauma can lead to feelings of isolation and disconnection from others. During the traumatic event, we may have needed to feel connected to others for comfort, reassurance, and support.

3.  Empowerment: During the traumatic event, we may have felt powerless and helpless, and we needed to regain a sense of control and agency to protect ourselves from harm and danger.

4. Validation: During the traumatic event, we may have felt like our experiences were being invalidated or dismissed, and we needed to be heard and acknowledged by others to feel validated and understood.

5. Meaning-making: During the traumatic event, we may have struggled to make sense of what was happening and needed to understand the situation and its impact on us to cope with the experience.

6. Boundaries: During the traumatic event, our boundaries may have been crossed or blurred, and we needed to assert our boundaries to protect ourselves from further harm.

7. Trust: During the traumatic event, our trust in ourselves, others, and the world around us may have been shaken, and we needed to rely on ourselves or others we trusted to feel safe and secure.

8. Emotional support: Trauma can be emotionally overwhelming, and we may have needed emotional support from others to cope with the intense feelings during the traumatic event.

9. Physical care: Depending on the nature of the trauma, we may have had physical needs that required immediate attention and care during the traumatic event, such as medical attention or safety equipment.

10. Stability: During the traumatic event, our lives may have been uprooted and destabilized, and we needed to find ways to create stability and routine to help us feel grounded.

11. Expression: Trauma can be difficult to articulate, and we may have needed opportunities to express our thoughts and feelings about what was happening during and after the traumatic event.

12. Justice: If the traumatic event involved harm caused by another person or a violation of our rights, we may have needed justice or accountability to feel heard, acknowledged, valued, and safe.

13. Innocence: Trauma can shatter our sense of innocence and leave us feeling like the world is a dangerous and unpredictable place. It can also pressure us to grow up too soon. During the trauma, we may have needed to protect our innocence and sense of trust in others.

14. Sense of safety in the world: Trauma can erode our sense of safety in the world, leaving us feeling like nowhere is truly safe. During the trauma, we may have needed to find ways to feel safe and secure in our environment and with the people around us.

As you work through your *Heart Journey*™ *Journal Heartwork*, be sure to meet the need in every slice of trauma under the "What resource do you want here?" section. Use the above list as your guide.

## IT IS OVER

In our trauma work, we will start by acknowledging that the trauma is over. Identifying when the trauma ended is crucial because it provides a sense of closure and completion for the traumatic experience. Beloved, trauma can leave our brain stuck in a state of hyperarousal, constantly searching for potential threats and dangers. Recognizing when the trauma ended helps the brain differentiate between the past traumatic event and the present, which can help to shift out of the hyper-aroused state. This process also reduces the intensity of traumatic memories, making it easier to work through them. Acknowledging the trauma is over is empowering because it restores a sense of agency and control. It enables individuals to recognize that they have survived the traumatic event and can move forward in their healing journey.

# TIME REVERSE TRAUMA™ OVERVIEW

We will be using the Time Reverse Trauma™ Tool in your *Heart Journey*™ *Journal*, beginning with your least traumatic event. The process for each trauma is as follows: First, you will provide a detailed description of the trauma to open up the Memory Reconsolidation window. Second, you will identify when you knew the trauma was over, reminding your brain that the trauma is indeed over. Third, you will explore what it feels like in your body to know that the trauma is over. Fourth, you will choose an image that represents the end of the trauma to use in our trauma work. Fifth, you will identify who you desire to be with you, using your holy imagination, during this memory work, to ensure that you do not feel alone and have all the support you need. Sixth, you will work through the trauma, starting from T-7 and moving to T+7. For each block, you will describe what happened, identify the resources you would like to help you through it, and identify the responses you need to complete regarding fight, flight, orienting, etc.

To begin, we will start with the shallow end of pain regarding your traumas. We will not begin with traumas that are too overwhelming, and you will use Distancing Strategies as needed throughout. For instance, you can imagine memories flipped up on a movie screen or view them through Binoculars Backwards™, so they are more distant. When working on your trauma, consider having at least one foot in the present, and one foot in the past. Think of your body as being approximately 60 percent in the present and 40 percent in the past to add perspective. As you progress, you will become whole and move forward toward pursuing your purpose with a strong heart home. Much joy is before you, Beloved. Your prayer will shift from "Heal me, Lord" to "Use me, Lord. What is my assignment?"

## DEBORAH'S STORY

Deborah's use of the Time Reverse Trauma™ method allowed her to confront and overcome past traumas, including one of her earliest memories of physical and emotional abuse by her mother. This traumatic incident occurred when Deborah's mother violently slapped her across the face in front of her best friend, leaving her feeling confused and frightened. Deborah had been innocently playing with her best friend before the incident. The situation was exacerbated by the fact that Deborah's mother was rarely affectionate toward her, and Deborah already felt rejected. The slap left her feeling even more dejected, as if she had done something wrong, even though she could not understand why she was stricken.

As a result of the incident, Deborah's best friend ran away, and Deborah was left feeling embarrassed, confused, and ashamed. It was not until later that she learned that her friend had been afraid of Deborah's mother all along. This knowledge compounded Deborah's feelings of guilt and shame, leaving her feeling scared and alone. However, when she saw her friend smiling and moving toward her to chat the following Monday at school, Deborah felt a sense of relief and peace knowing that their friendship was still intact.

Deborah worked through each piece of this trauma, adding in all the support and encounters with Jesus that she needed. She also allowed unmet responses, such as running away from her mother and after her friend, to be completed using her holy imagination. Deborah experienced a great sense of relief after following these steps and felt a new settled feeling in her nervous system. She also experienced more safety with Jesus, imagining Him helping her mother be more kind. Let us use Deborah's experience as encouragement as we go through the Time Reverse Trauma™ Steps.

## TIME REVERSE TRAUMA™ STEPS

You will work in your *Heart Journey*™ *Journal* following these steps for each trauma. Get out your *Heart Journey*™ *Journal* and follow along as we go through these steps in **Individual Heartwork - Time Reverse Trauma**™. Then you will work through your traumas one at a time in your *Heart Journey*™ *Journal*.

1.  Begin by thinking of a milder trauma to start with, and we will go through these steps with each trauma. For instance, Deborah started with her mom slapping her and gradually moved up to more challenging traumas like her father's suicide.

2.  Bring the trauma to mind with curiosity and self-compassion, while connecting with Jesus and knowing He is with you, holding you.

3.  Once you identify the trauma, write down the moment when you knew it was over and you began to have a sense of things returning to normal. This moment is T+7 in our sequence. Ask yourself, "When did I feel a sense of relief like it was over?" For Deborah, she knew the trauma was over when she saw her best friend on Monday and was assured that their friendship was still intact.

4.  Remember the sense of relief at the moment you knew it was over. Focus on what that felt like in your body and try to identify an image you can keep coming back to, to remind yourself that it is over. See Jesus in this moment, holding you, filling you, reassuring you. Examples of such moments could be seeing a loved one after the event, coming home from the hospital, or moving out of a toxic environment. Bringing this moment forward experientially, feeling relief, is important for your nervous system. Write down your experience and create a relieving image you can revisit to remind yourself that the trauma is over. For instance, Deborah wrote, "I feel relief as I

remember my best friend's smiling face. I feel relief in my body and connection to my best friend, like ties between us that are strong. I see Jesus standing behind her, reassuring me that He is with me." Then Deborah drew a picture of the happy smiling face of her friend with the smiling face of Jesus behind her.

5.  Take some time and write down who you would have liked to have with you during the trauma. This person or entity could be anyone from Jesus and angels to a spouse, pet, or close friend. Imagine them being there with you, loving you, meeting every need. Soften into the support as much as you can with your holy imagination, know God never intended for you to be wounded and alone. Imagine them being present with you in the moment of the trauma, helping and supporting you. Add as many supports and helps in as you want, the more the better. You can also bring in Self as Mom. Deborah imagined Jesus being with her as well as angels, stopping her mother's hand and helping her mother to perceive how lovable Deborah was. She also used Self-Momming™ to comfort and validate her younger part. Use your holy imagination to see and feel each need being met.

6.  Next, work through the timeline of the trauma one slice at a time. Work your way through in this order: T-7, T-6, T-5, T-4, T-3, T-2, T-1, T=0, T+1, T+2, T+3, T+4, T+5, T+6, T+7 with T standing for Trauma. T-7 represents when everything was okay, right before you were alerted to something being wrong. T+7 represents when you knew the trauma was over. Start at T -7 when everything was okay before the event, and write or draw what was happening at the time. For each slice of the trauma, work through the following steps:

    a.  Remember the moment in the slice of time with which you are working. Look around with your five senses and remember what you saw, heard, smelt, tasted, and touched. Remember what you thought. In this way, you open the

Memory Reconsolidation Window for changing emotional learning.

b. Identify the resources you needed at the slice time you are processing. These can be people, the Lord, or any type of help or intervention. Make sure you meet your need in the moment. Imagine what resources could help you in that moment. In this way, we are creating the Prediction Error for change in emotional learning. Write them down. Deborah wrote down, "Jesus, angels, and Self as Mom."

c. As you feel sensations in your body, track them and imagine being able to complete any unresolved nervous system response (orienting, defensive responding, fight, flight). In this way, we are continuing to create a Prediction Error for change in emotional learning, and we are also discharging the pent up trauma from the body. Write down the completed nervous system response that you need. If it is too much, slow down the work or contact your group facilitator, accountability or prayer partner, or a professional licensed psychotherapist. Deborah wrote down, "I am able to run away from my mother while Jesus takes care of her and get to run to my friend's house where it is safe."

d. Use Distancing Strategies as needed to stay within the Window of Tolerance while still making sure you feel the impact of the event to open the Memory Reconciliation Window. Take breaks as needed. In this way, we are staying in the areas of your brain and nervous system where change in emotional learning can occur. Deborah imagined the event playing on a movie screen at T=0 to make the hardest part of the trauma more manageable and to enable her remaining in the Window of Tolerance.

e. Write everything down to help encode this new learning.

f. Move to the next slice of time.

g.   Move through to the end of the memory (T+7)

## DEBORAH'S SLICE SEQUENCE

Deborah worked through these slices: playing happily with my best friend (T-7); mom calling me with an angry voice (T-6); feeling shame over how mom says my name so angrily (T-5); looking at my friend in fear (T-4); running to mom in the dining room (T-3); seeing mom's rage-filled eyes (T-2); watching mom raise her hand (T-1); feeling the sting of a slap across my face (T=0); feeling shocked and alarmed (T+1); flooded with confusion and shame as mom yells at me (T+2); crocodile tears flow from my eyes and I blush with more shame, hoping my friend did not see or hear (T+3); mom keeps yelling at me as I stand there stunned, not understanding what she is saying. I give up on being understood by mom. (T+4); I run to find my friend, desperately searching all over the house (T+5); I run outside to look for her to no avail (T+6); and, I see my friend's smiling face the next day at school (T+7).

Now it is your turn, Beloved!

Complete **Individual Heartwork - Time Reverse Trauma**™ within your *Heart Journey*™ *Journal* at this time.

## STICKY MEMORIES

We will now look for Sticky Memories that still feel unresolved after our Time Reverse Trauma™ work, in the same manner that we used in Chapter Six of our study.

Complete **Individual Heartwork - Sticky Memories** within your *Heart Journey*™ *Journal* Chapter Seven, at this time.

## TOOLS FOR STICKY TRAUMAS

Similar to the previous chapter, we will use several tools for working with Sticky Memories, all of which have their foundation in our faith in Jesus and use Memory Reconsolidation. We will use Oscillation with Jesus™, Pain to Purpose Drawing™, and The Beautiful Place Prayer™.

## OSCILLATION WITH JESUS™

We will re-use our Oscillation with Jesus™ tool to resolve Sticky Memories that feel unresolved after your Time Reverse Trauma™ work. Oscillation involves following an imaginary figure-eight with a positive and negative stimulus associated with the trauma, in order to integrate new, positive emotional learning into the memory and reduce emotional distress. Refer to Chapter Six of the study for directions for the Oscillation with Jesus™ technique.

Complete **Individual Heartwork - Oscillation with Jesus™** within your *Heart Journey™ Journal* Chapter Seven, at this time.

Use this QR code to access audible versions of activities.

## PAIN TO PURPOSE DRAWING™

To help with unresolved Sticky Memories, the Pain to Purpose Drawing™ tool can be used for trauma memories, similar to our use for unmet need memories in Chapter Six. This tool involves drawing three pictures related to the memory—the first depicting the felt sense of the trauma memory, the second the opposite feeling, and the third drawing what the Lord wants to create with the pain to transform it into a Beautiful Place through the Heart Journey Beautiful Place Prayer™. This prayer involves surrendering the pain to God and asking Him to turn it into something beautiful, trusting that He will work all things together for good. By using Pneumaception™, we can hear what the Lord wants to do with the pain and draw what He shows, experiencing hope and Kingdom purpose. For more information on Pain to Purpose Drawing™, refer to Chapter Six.

Complete **Individual Heartwork - Pain to Purpose Drawing™** within your *Heart Journey™ Journal* Chapter Seven, at this time.

## BEAUTIFUL PLACE PRAYER™

We will also use the Beautiful Place Prayer™ in this chapter to write our explicit prayers over each trauma, praying for the Lord to make each a beautiful place. This prayer is my "go to" when I encounter trials. Once I realize I must walk through a fiery difficulty, I determine to trust God to use it for His glory and to help others. He has never let me down, and He will not let you down. As Romans 8:28 (NIV) says, "And we know that in all things God works for the good of those who love Him, who have been called according to His purpose."

Complete **Individual Heartwork - Beautiful Place Prayer™** within your *Heart Journey™ Journal* Chapter Seven, at this time.

## GRIEF AND TRAUMA

As we work through our traumas, it is important to remember that the tools we learned in Chapter Six about processing losses and uncovered grief can also be applied here. Leaning into God's love and comfort, scheduling time to process our feelings, and practicing self-compassion are essential tools for navigating the emotional journey of trauma work. Writing letters to our inner child after doing inner child work can also provide comfort and aid in healing. It is important to remember that healing takes time, and seeking support from trusted sources is always an option. By using a combination of faith and psychological skills, we can find peace and wholeness.

## FAMILY LINE WORK

The story of Gideon in the book of Judges serves as an important reminder of the need to address any family idols or sins that may hinder our ability to fulfill our calling and purpose in life. Gideon's act of obedience in tearing down the altar of Baal and the Asherah pole that his own father had built, cleared the way for him to fulfill his calling as a leader and deliverer of the Israelites.

Similarly, we may need to address any family idols or sins that are hindering us from fulfilling our purpose and calling. This may involve identifying and breaking patterns of behavior that have been passed down through generations. By doing so, we can invite God to work in our lives and use us for His purposes.

Research has shown that trauma and sins can be passed down through genetics, as well as family history.[26] It is important to reflect on our family's heritage and genetic line and invite God into these spaces to reverse any trauma that may still be affecting us. By calling upon the Holy Spirit and breaking patterns of generational sin, we can move forward with freedom and healing.

To begin this process, we can write down any sins or traumas that we are aware of in our family line in our *Heart Journey*™ *Journal Heartwork*. We can reflect on the experiences of our family members and recognize the impact of these issues on ourselves and our loved ones. Then we can prayerfully ask for forgiveness for the sins of our fathers and forefathers and pray for healing for the traumas that have affected our families.

This type of prayer is best done in a Heart Group or with an accountability partner. In Matthew 18:18-20, Jesus reminds us that when two or three gather in His name, He is with them. The Bible reflects that there is power in coming together for prayer in numbers (2 Chronicles 6:34-35; 1 Thessalonians 5:25). We are authorized to bind up curses and loose blessings (Matthew 16:19). Therefore, we can agree in prayer with others and invite God to work in our lives and our families. By prayerfully breaking the cycle of generational sin and trauma, we can find freedom and restoration and fulfill our purpose without hindrance from legacy burdens.

Complete **Individual Heartwork - Family Line Work** within your *Heart Journey*™ *Journal* Chapter Seven, at this time.

## MOVING FORWARD

As we conclude this chapter, I want to take a moment to acknowledge all the hard work you have completed so far. You have learned and practiced valuable RESOURCE™ skills, made positive changes to your negative habits, created your timelines, Satisfied Unmet Needs™, and Time Reversed Traumas™. Chapters Six and Seven were undoubtedly challenging, and I want you to know that I am incredibly proud of you for persevering and showing up for yourself and Jesus in this way. Can you feel your heart home healing?

Just as the dilapidated areas of a cottage undergo reconstruction and transformation to become beautiful and functional, so, too, are you undergoing a process of healing and transformation. And just as the reconstruction of a cottage can be a difficult and messy process, your journey toward healing has been challenging at times. But always remember that just as the end result of a reconstructed cottage is a beautiful and cozy home, the end result of your healing journey will be a beautiful and whole-hearted life. Keep up the good work, and know that I am here on these pages to support you every step of the way.

Moving forward, we will be focusing on healing our boundaries in Chapter Eight. This is an essential step in our journey to wholeness and self-love. Through setting and maintaining healthy boundaries, we can protect ourselves from further harm, build stronger relationships, and live a more authentic life in Jesus. As always, we will be using a combination of faith and psychological tools to support the growth and healing of your heart home. Remember to be gentle with yourself and take things at your own pace. You are worthy of love and care, and I believe in your ability to heal and thrive.

You are pursuing healing so fiercely, Beloved. You are at the half-way mark of this noble journey! Be sure to finish your **Individual Heartwork - Chapter Seven Review** and your **Heart Group Discussion** work with your small group or with a friend. In the next chapter, we work with Jesus to heal our boundaries!

## LET US PRAY.

*Heavenly Father,*

*We give You all our trauma, and we trust that You are turning every trauma into a blessing. You turn our ashes into beauty. It was one of Your first promises at the beginning of Your ministry, that You heal the brokenhearted and turn our ashes into beauty. We give You these ashes and pray that You would come into every area of our hearts and heal mightily. We pray that You would pull every bit of trauma out of places in our minds where it is stuck, that You would integrate into healthy spaces, and that You would soak Your Spirit into each place. Thank You that You Time Reversed™ all our trauma! Lord, I thank You that my trauma is*

Time Reversed™ and that the enemy can no longer use trauma or the effects of it against me. In Jesus' name, I speak that I am free from every impact of trauma.

Lord, regarding the sins of our forefathers, we ask that You forgive. We confess these things as sin (name each one out loud). I ask that You forgive my whole family line. Lord, I repent on behalf of my forefathers. (Name those things and ask the Lord to cover them). And Lord, we claim that Your blood covers every sin. We break the curse of where the enemy has been able to work through these family sins. We break the curse of all traumas that have been passed down. God, we break the genetic curse of traumas passed down before us. (Name the trauma). Thank You that the enemy has no place in my family.

Now we move forward in that new freedom with nothing from the past holding us back. We believe we are free in Jesus' name, based on Your finished work in the cross and resurrection. You have already transformed us so much on this beautiful, healing Heart Journey™. Thank You, Father.

Please continue Your good work, bringing us closer to You each day. May our hearts and minds continue to be open to Your renovations, and may we recognize where You are working in our lives. We pray that You would fill us with Your love, joy, and peace, and that we would continue to grow in our faith, hope, and trust in You. Lord, we pray for protection from the enemy, and that You would cover us with Your precious blood and shield us from harm.

We thank You, Lord, for Your grace and mercy, and for Your faithfulness to us. We give You all the praise, honor, and glory.

In Jesus' name, Amen.

# *Chapter*

## EIGHT

### Restoring My Boundaries

*Let your Yes be simply Yes, and your No be simply No; anything more than that comes from the evil one.*

**Matthew 5:37 (AMPC)**

As we continue with our RECONSTRUCTION™ acronym, we are at "R" which stands for "Repair Boundary Ruptures." In this chapter, we will discover what boundaries are and how God operates through boundaries. We will define our boundaries, and discover how to live from "true self" and empowerment. In addition, we will uncover areas in our lives where our boundaries have been ruptured and facilitate healing through encounters with Jesus in those places. Last, we will learn to set personal boundaries without false guilt.

## IMPACT OF BOUNDARIES

In the natural world, we establish physical boundaries around our homes, businesses, and cars to protect our possessions. We lock our doors, put up fences, and password protect private information. It is equally important to have strong and healthy personal boundaries in our relational lives. When our personal boundaries are crossed, we may experience feelings of being used, wounded, unheard, or disrespected in our hearts.

To better understand the impact of boundary encroachments, imagine a scenario where a neighbor continues to help themselves to items in your kitchen without your consent, but where you also have never voiced a limit. Over time, your neighbor's behavior continues and escalates, due to lack of limits set. They begin to use your toiletries, borrow your car, and even move into your spare bedroom. If this pattern persists, how might this affect your relationship with your neighbor? How might you feel about yourself for allowing it? Would you experience resentment and bitterness toward your neighbor? Furthermore, how might this situation impact the character of both parties involved?

While this analogy may seem extreme, it accurately depicts the consequences of boundary ruptures in relationships. We often say "yes" when we really mean "no," or we say "no" when we really mean "yes." Other times, we expect others to read our minds, and when they fail to do so, we harbor resentment toward them. On the flip side, we might also discover that we have been inadvertently taking advantage of others without fully owning accountability for our own lives. We allow others to do for us that which we should be doing for ourselves. In either case, both parties must learn to responsibly steward their own boundaries.

## WHAT IS A BOUNDARY?

A boundary is an imaginary line that separates us from others and defines our personal space, beliefs, values, and the way we interact with others. A boundary delineates who we are as an individual, what we need, with whom we will or will not engage, and what we will tolerate within relationships and within ourselves.

Boundaries are our inheritance as daughters of God, as we have all been given a self to steward. The self is defined by boundaries, which are essential to showing up as the unique one-time event that you are in the world. There will never be another you, but if you fail to show up with healthy boundaries, the world cannot really see the beauty of you, defined.

Boundaries are foundational to trust-building in relationships. When we make the effort to understand and respect another person's boundaries, it allows us to know and trust them better, thus fostering a deeper connection.

Boundaries are volitional and must be spoken and enforced by us. No one can do this for us. When we live without boundaries, others cannot quite make out who we are because we are not defining ourselves for them. For true and authentic relationships to thrive, it is crucial for both parties to communicate and respect each other's "yes" and "no."

## SAYING "NO"

One key aspect of healthy boundaries is the ability to say "no" when necessary. Saying no can be difficult, especially if we are used to people pleasing or have a fear of conflict. However, saying no is an important protection for our well-being. It is key to remember that saying no does not make us selfish or unkind, but rather, allows us to properly prioritize our needs and values.

In contrast, weak or unhealthy boundaries can lead to a range of negative outcomes. For example, we may find ourselves feeling overwhelmed, anxious, or resentful in our relationships. We may struggle to assert ourselves or communicate our needs effectively, leading to a sense of powerlessness. We may also find ourselves attracting people who do not respect our boundaries or who take advantage of us. Boundary crossers and those with blurry boundaries tend to find each other like positive and negative sides of magnets.

## YOUR BRAIN IS MADE FOR BOUNDARIES

Many of us struggle with boundary setting, but be encouraged that your brain is structured for boundaries! For instance, the somatosensory cortex and the insula cortex work together to keep us informed of that which we are experiencing in our bodies and emotions, enabling us to determine what feels appropriate or inappropriate for us. Meanwhile, the basal forebrain system plays a crucial role in emotional resonance and empathy, helping us understand the needs of others and setting boundaries that respect both their needs and ours. By paying attention to these internal cues, we can set boundaries that align with our values and attune to our and others' needs.

Furthermore, our frontal and parietal lobes, including our mirror neurons, are critical in resonating with others and comprehending their perspective. This ability is essential for establishing healthy boundaries. Moreover, our HPA system is a regulatory organization that releases cortisol when we encounter stressors, which can help us identify when our boundaries are being violated. Finally, the tenth cranial nerve, the vagus nerve, is responsible for relaxation and deactivating our stress response when we feel secure and connected to others. By attuning to the sensations produced by these structures, we can develop awareness regarding our intrapersonal and interpersonal boundaries and make choices that prioritize our overall well-being. What does all this mean for us as women of God? God made you for boundary-setting!

## BOUNDARIES ARE NOT ...

As we strive to identify what healthy boundaries are, it is important to understand what boundaries are not. Boundaries are not a way to control others (as much as we would sometimes like to!). We must avoid the temptation to control or manipulate others to get our desired outcome or to avoid pain. We communicate how we will or will not respond to the actions of others, but we avoid attempting to control.

In addition, we need to consider that God wants people to reap what they sow as a learning mechanism (Galatians 6:7-8). This means that at times, we need to allow natural consequences to unfold in the lives of others, even when it is demanding or painful to watch. Boundaries should not be about doing for others what they can do for themselves or covering up for their mistakes. We should not suffer because of other people's actions by paying their consequences for them. And we should not allow ourselves to be used or abused in the interest of helping others. Remember that we are designed to be led by the Spirit of God, not by fear, false guilt, or people pleasing (Romans 8:14).

For example, Sarah has a young adult son who struggles with drug addiction. Instead of setting clear boundaries with her son, she constantly bails him out of jail, and covers up for his mistakes financially. She feels desperately afraid of seeing him in jail, or worse. However, Sarah's enabling behavior is preventing her son from experiencing the consequences of his actions and learning from them. Her behavior is disrupting the law of sowing and reaping and is inadvertently enabling her son to continue his destructive behavior. As a result, Sarah's son is not taking responsibility for his actions. By bowing to fear, Sarah has ceased following the leading of the Spirit and has disrupted God's law of sowing and reaping.

## DAILY AND EXCESSIVE BURDENS

"What about carrying each other's burdens?" you might ask. In Galatians 6:2, the Greek word used for carrying each other's "burdens" is "baros," which refers to a heavy or oppressive burden that is too difficult to bear alone. This verse encourages believers to carry each other's excessive burdens. In contrast, Galatians 6:5 says we should each carry our own load. The Greek word used for "load" is "phortion," which refers to a burden that is more manageable and individual. This verse teaches us that each person should carry their own load. In essence, these two Scriptures together state that we should each carry our daily "backpack" and help each other through seasons of excessive stress. Understanding the difference between "baros" and "phortion" can help us avoid taking on burdens that are not ours to bear while taking responsibility for our own load.

Complete **Individual Heartwork - Daily and Excessive Burdens** within your *Heart Journey*™ *Journal* at this time.

## TRUE AND FALSE SELF

When we strive to live in healthy boundaries by the Spirit of God, we are discovering how to live from our "true selves," created by God. The true self is the core of who God made us to be, our deepest and purest desires, passions, longings, values, thoughts, inclinations, expressions, and beliefs. It is the authentic self that reflects the unique image of God within us.

On the other hand, the false self is a mask we wear out of fear. The false self can manifest in various ways, such as people pleasing, perfectionism, and codependency. It is not a reflection of who we truly are, but rather a defense mechanism to protect ourselves from pain and rejection. The false self is a product of our past experiences, traumas, and societal pressures that have shaped our beliefs and behaviors about how to show up "acceptably."

Identifying and embracing our true selves can be challenging, especially if we have experienced trauma or have adopted a "false self" for a long time. Nonetheless, we are called to live an authentic life that reflects the image of Christ within us. As stated in Romans 12:2 (ESV), "Do not be conformed to this world, but be transformed by the renewal of your mind, that by testing you may discern what is the will of God, what is good and acceptable and perfect."

Living in the "true self" requires tolerating a level of differentiation from others. Differentiation refers to the ability to maintain a sense of individuality and independence within relationships, while connection refers to the ability to remain emotionally close and engaged with others. Both are needed to show up as your true self in relationships.

Complete **Individual Heartwork - True and False Self** within your *Heart Journey*™ *Journal* at this time.

## GOD'S BOUNDARIES

Have you ever considered that God operates within boundaries? As Christian women, we may sometimes feel that giving all we have to every request is the best way to emulate God's love. However, when we look to God's Word, we see that He has strong boundaries.

For instance, He articulates what He likes and dislikes. In Exodus 20:3-17, God gives the Israelites the Ten Commandments, which are a clear set of boundaries for how to live a life that pleases Him. Similarly, in Deuteronomy 6:5-9, He commands His people to love Him with all their heart, soul, and strength, and to teach His commandments to their children. In Proverbs 6:16-19, He lists seven things He hates, including haughty eyes, a lying tongue, and hands that shed innocent blood. In Isaiah 61:8, He declares that He loves justice and hates robbery and wrongdoing. And in Deuteronomy 28, He shares the consequences of obedience and disobedience.

In addition, throughout the Scriptures, God also tells us who He is and is not. For example, in Psalm 103:8-14, He reveals Himself as a compassionate and merciful God, but He is also a just God who will not let sin go unpunished (Romans 6:23). In Isaiah 45:5-7, He proclaims Himself as the only true God and the Creator of all things. Moreover, God tells us how to enter into relationship with Him. In John 14:6 (NIV), Jesus says, "I am the way and the truth and the life. No one comes to the Father except through me."

Boundaries are good. They originated with God. As we are made in the Father's image, we are designed to operate within strong and clear boundaries.

## DEFINING MY BOUNDARIES

Before we can operate within boundaries, we must define our boundaries. Boundaries can be defined via our use of personal space, physical distance, words, values, actions, limits, choices, gifts and resources, thoughts, passions, attitudes, emotional distance, and external extensions of ourselves. We will explore each of the areas as we seek to define our own boundaries. As you look over these areas, consider the state of your own boundaries. Then you will engage in written reflections on these areas in your *Heart Journey*™ *Journal.*

1.  Values: Our values can guide our decisions and help us stay true to ourselves and our faith. (Joshua 24:15) Example: "I am sorry, but I cannot participate in that activity as it goes against my values and beliefs."

2.  Words: We can use our words to express our thoughts and feelings in a clear and respectful manner, while also setting boundaries when necessary. (Proverbs 15:1, Ephesians 4:15) Example: "I appreciate your concern, but I am not comfortable discussing this topic with you."

3.  Actions and Behaviors: Our actions and behaviors can communicate our boundaries to others and help us stay consistent in our beliefs and values. (1 Corinthians 10:31) Example: "I choose not to steal office supplies because it goes against my personal beliefs and values."

4.  Limits: Setting limits on our time, energy, and resources can help us avoid burnout and maintain healthy relationships. (Ecclesiastes 3:1-8) Example: "I can only commit to volunteering once a week as I have other responsibilities to attend to."

5.  Choices: We can make intentional choices about how we spend our time, who we spend it with, and what we invest our resources in. (Proverbs 3:6) Example: "I am choosing to prioritize my family and spend less than fifteen minutes a day on social media."

6.  Thoughts: We can set boundaries on our thought life by choosing to focus on positive, uplifting thoughts and avoiding destructive thinking patterns. (Philippians 4:8) Example: "I am not going to dwell on the negative aspects of this situation, but instead, I will focus on the positive character traits and intimacy with Jesus I am developing within this trial."

7.  Attitudes: Our attitudes can influence how we approach the world and relationships, and how we set boundaries with others. (Colossians 3:12-14) Example: "I will choose to approach this situation with love and kindness, but I will also set boundaries to protect my emotional well-being."

8.  Personal Space: We can show our boundaries by setting aside time for ourselves to rest, recharge, and reflect on our relationship with God. (Mark 6:31) Example: "I am taking Sunday afternoon to rest and spend time with God, so I will not be available for any other commitments."

9.  Physical Distance: We can maintain physical distance from people who may not have our best interests at heart, or who may be harmful to our spiritual, emotional, or physical well-being. (Proverbs 22:24-25) Example: "I am not comfortable being alone with you, so I will only meet in public places."

10. Passions: We can give ourselves fully to passions that align with our values and priorities, while setting boundaries on those that may be harmful or distract us from our relationship with God. (1 Corinthians 6:12) Example: "I am passionate about fitness, but I will not compromise my commitment to attend church on Sundays."

11. Stewarding of our Gifts/Talents: We can use our unique God-given gifts and talents to serve others while also setting boundaries on our time and energy. (1 Peter 4:10) Example: "I am willing to use my graphic design skills to create a flyer for the event, but I cannot attend the meeting as it conflicts with my schedule."

12. Stewarding of our Resources: We can be good stewards of our financial resources by setting boundaries on our spending and investing in things that align with our values and priorities. (Luke 16:11) Example: "I have set a budget for myself and cannot afford to purchase that item at this time."

13. Emotional Distance: Sometimes, we may need to create emotional distance from people who are not supportive or who may be harmful to our spiritual or emotional well-being. (2 Corinthians 6:14) Example: "I need some space right now to process my feelings, so I will not be responding to messages or calls for a while."

14. External Extensions of Me: Fences/barriers around our things can be a physical representation of our boundaries and can help us protect our possessions and maintain healthy relationships. (Proverbs 22:3) Example: "I have put a lock on

my personal belongings to protect them, and I ask that you respect my boundaries by not using or borrowing them without my permission."

Complete **Individual Heartwork - Defining My Boundaries** within your *Heart Journey*™ *Journal* at this time.

## YOUR VOICE

Beloved, after defining your boundaries, you must voice them. When we were children, it was our parents' role to draw out and honor our voices and ensure our needs were voiced and met. Now, as adults, we are responsible for volitionally voicing our needs. Maintaining healthy boundaries requires clear verbal statements on what we need and what we will and will not do, give, and be around. No matter how difficult, we must practice stewarding our voice by using it in our relationships.

Communicating healthy boundaries enables us to preserve and manage our heart homes while also creating space for others. If we do not assert our boundaries, we will unwisely morph into the wills of others. God desires for us to "connect" with others rather than "merge" with others, and this requires wisely expressing your true self. In addition, we must remember that healthy boundaries also require voicing consent and respecting others' consent or non-consent.

## THE LAW OF ENTROPY

The law of entropy, the will of others, and the unseen spiritual war in which we live, all work as resistance to godly boundaries. The law of entropy, also known as the second law of thermodynamics, is a fundamental principle in physics that states that the total entropy, or disorder, of an isolated system will always increase over time. In simpler terms, the law of entropy can be understood as the tendency for things to become disordered or chaotic over time, unless energy is continuously put into the system to maintain order. The law of entropy explains that if we do not exert energy into boundary setting, our boundaries and our relationships will naturally decay and break down.

Boundary entropy occurs because the needs, desires, and wills of others around us often press on us. The needs and wants of others will infringe upon on our own boundaries if we do not take a loving, but assertive stance. If we do not delineate our boundaries, the will of others will define how we live and act in the world, and we will live as people pleasers. Often, this is not malicious on the part of others, but occurs when we omit putting up a fence to define our boundaries. Think about two countries, living side by side. Without a clear boundary line, it would be easy for encroachment on either side. Paul said in Galatians 1:10 (NIV), "If I were still trying to please man, I would not be a servant of Christ." When we set boundaries, we step out of people pleasing and into our true selves, created for His glory.

In addition, we know that we live in an unseen spiritual war where the enemy wants to move us out of true self and out of the will of God. Hence, we need to establish and maintain clear boundaries in our daily lives to prevent the enemy's advancement in our lives. Scripture says, "Be alert and of sober mind. Your enemy the devil prowls around like a roaring lion looking for someone to devour" (1 Peter 5:8, NIV).

For example, without good boundaries in place, we may allow people to take advantage of us and then become resentful. Suppose Chalice has a friend who frequently asks for money but never pays her back. She needs to set a boundary by saying "no" when the friend asks her for money in the future. If she continues to lend the friend money without setting a boundary, the friend will continue to take advantage of her. Chalice might develop feelings of resentment, frustration, and even bitterness toward the friend, and then the enemy has a stronghold within Chalice (Ephesians 4:26-27). By setting a boundary, Chalice would protect herself from being taken advantage of and show the other person that she values her own resources and is not willing to be used. By applying healthy boundaries, we can be good stewards of all that God has given us and resist the law of entropy.

## STEPPING OFF THE TRIANGLE OF PAIN

The Triangle of Pain, also called the Karpman Drama Triangle, is a model that illustrates three interconnected roles—victim, persecutor, and rescuer—commonly seen in relationships with boundary issues. It highlights how power struggles and dysfunctional dynamics can emerge when individuals struggle to establish healthy boundaries and engage in harmful patterns of interaction. When we find ourselves caught in these roles, we often experience a sense of entrapment, powerlessness, and growing resentment within the relational dynamic. When we are on the Triangle of Pain, we are usually not just reacting to the person in front of us, but also to unmet needs and trauma triggers from our past.

The persecutor is the person who blames, criticizes, or attacks the other, and wants the other to change so the persecutor can have her needs met. The victim is the person who feels powerless and helpless, often blaming themselves and others for their situation, and wants someone else to rescue her. The caretaker is the person who tries to rescue and fix others, often at the cost of their own well-being. These roles are often fluid like a reactive and interactive dance, with each party taking turns in differing roles. None of these roles promote healthy, adult-to-adult relationships, and all involve poor boundaries.

Often, we find ourselves getting pulled into the Triangle of Pain when we experience triggers in our relationships. It is common to feel a physical response, such as a rise in our nervous system or a twisting feeling in our abdomen, once we find ourselves on the Triangle. When we are on the Triangle of Pain, we can quickly switch positions, going round and round the triangle, while the person we are interacting with does the same.

The basic premise behind boundaries and empowered interactions is "I'm okay and can handle my daily load, and you're okay and can handle your daily load." But when we are on the Triangle, we stop relating as adults who can carry our own daily loads. On the Triangle, someone is always "not okay." The caretaker thinks, "I won't be okay until you're okay." The persecutor thinks, "You'll be okay as soon as you take my advice." And the victim thinks, "I won't be okay until you take care of me." The key to overcoming the Triangle of Pain is to step off of it and return to "I am okay, and you are okay." We take responsibility of our own daily lives, and trust that others can choose to do the same.

One way to break free from the Triangle of Pain is to focus on the Triangle of Empowerment. The Triangle of Empowerment has three roles: coach, challenger, and creator. These roles promote healthy adult-to-adult relationships and encourage personal growth and empowerment. The coach's role involves supporting and guiding others without rescuing them. The challenger role involves holding others accountable while respecting their autonomy. The creator role involves taking responsibility for one's own life and actively pursuing goals and dreams.

Complete **Individual Heartwork - Stepping off the Triangle of Pain** within your *Heart Journey*™ *Journal* at this time.

## PERSECUTION OR BOUNDARY ISSUE?

Occasionally, we are persecuted for the sake of Christ. Sharing in the sufferings of Christ can mean allowing ourselves to be insulted or mistreated in a certain way for the sake of Jesus. Yet, we are not going to choose to be in relationships like this outside of a specific call of God. I bring this up because at times women perceive that they are frequently being persecuted, but are actually over-spiritualizing a boundary problem. If you find yourself in a pattern of consistently being mistreated or abused in your relationships, this may be a sign that you need to evaluate and strengthen your boundaries.

On the other hand, some of us struggle with crossing others' boundaries and then receive negative feedback. In this case, the feedback is not persecution, but a natural consequence to our overstep. For instance, we may tend to transgress boundaries by sharing personal information or opinions without being invited to do so. It is important to recognize when we may be crossing boundaries and take steps to correct our behavior. This may involve apologizing to those we have hurt, asking for permission before sharing personal information, or simply being more aware of others' boundaries and respecting them.

Matthew 18:15-20 (NIV) provides a scriptural basis for setting boundaries in relationships through clear, non-manipulative verbal communication. Jesus instructs His disciples on how to handle conflict within the church community, emphasizing the importance of communication and reconciliation. In verse 15, He says, "If your brother or sister sins, go and point out their fault, just between the two of you. If they listen to you, you have won them over."

## MATCHING MY INNER AND RELATIONAL LIFE

When relating from a false self, we are suppressing our inner signals regarding what we are truly comfortable with. In an effort to listen to and live more pristinely within our boundaries, we will work on Matching My Inner and Relational Life in our Heartwork. This activity looks similar to our Socialgram™, but will be used differently. In your *Heart Journey™ Journal*, you will see two sets of concentric circles. You will measure how you are relating to others in reality, versus how your inner true self really feels toward those others.

Complete **Individual Heartwork - Matching My Inner and Relational Life** within your *Heart Journey™ Journal* at this time.

## RESTORED BOUNDARIES

Beloved, at this point in the chapter, you are likely aware of the need for repaired boundaries in your own life. Setting healthy boundaries involves identifying and expressing our wants and needs, and holding onto ourselves, others, and the Lord simultaneously. By staying connected to our inner selves, to others, and to God, we can make decisions based on all the relevant data. Ultimately, we want to follow the Lord in every situation.

Take time now to go to your *Heart Journey*™ *Journal* and complete the **Boundaries Restored Activity**.

Use this QR code to access audible versions of activities.

Wonderful work, Beloved. Jesus is indeed reconstructing your heart home! I believe He is deeply pleased with you, and so am I! Remember, we are not aiming for perfection, but forward movement. Next, we will work with your implicit somatic sense of boundaries, which will bring us back to some discussion of trauma.

## IMPLICIT BODILY MEMORY

When we interact with the world around us, our earthly five senses—sight, hearing, touch, taste, and smell—detect information and send it to our brain through sensory receptors. This sensory information is then processed by different parts of the brain, depending on the specific sense involved, and integrated with other neural signals to create a comprehensive understanding of our environment.

In the case of trauma, when a person experiences a particularly overwhelming or threatening event, the sensory information related to that event can enter the nervous system in a way that disrupts normal neural functioning. This can trigger a range of physical and psychological reactions, including feelings of fear, anxiety, and dissociation. These reactions can be particular to certain areas of the body, and can become embedded in long-term implicit bodily memory. This means that implicit somatic memory of trauma can be stored in the body at a semi-conscious sensory and emotional level, rather than just as a conscious memory.

Implicit somatic memory is a crucial concept in understanding the relationship between boundaries and the body. Trauma can be held in the body as somatic memory, which can impact our behavior and emotional responses. In situations where our boundaries have been violated, our bodies may hold onto those memories and manifest them as physical sensations when we are in similar situations in the present.[27] This can make it challenging to set and maintain healthy boundaries, as our body may be signaling us to respond in a certain way based on past experiences.

To cultivate healthy boundaries, it is important to understand our somatic and implicit felt sense in the 360 degree quadrant around and within our bodies. This involves becoming aware of the physical sensations and feelings that arise when we are in different situations or around different people. By tuning into our body's signals, we can start to identify patterns and triggers that may be related to past experiences.

Moreover, we want to welcome Jesus into every part of our bodily experience to bring restoration.

Jesus, our compassionate Shepherd, finds great delight in the restoration of what was once lost. In Luke 15, He shares three parables—the lost sheep, the lost coin, and the prodigal son—to highlight His immense joy when recovering that which was missing. Likewise, His desire is for every aspect of your heart and embodied existence to find refuge and healing in His loving embrace, returning home to the safety and wholeness found only in Him.

## DEBORAH'S STORY

Deborah's past traumas of being chased and whipped out of her father's rage had left her with a hypersensitivity to being approached from behind. When she worked through her *Heart Journey*™ *Journal* work, she identified a strong sense of vulnerability in her lower back, as if someone were coming up behind her. She also realized she was easily startled when others approached her from behind. This sensitivity was likely an implicit boundary rupture from her past that encoded through the sense of touch (being hit), sight (seeing her father ragefully chasing her), and sound (her father's angry voice behind her, and the sound of being hit). Through her *Heart Journey*™ work, she softened into more of the safety of Jesus in her body, and welcomed Jesus into the memories associated with her body's memories.

## 360 QUADRANT EXERCISE

In this segment of our study, we will engage in *Heart Journey*™ work in your journal that deepens your somatic healing from trauma. We will identify areas of implicit somatic boundary ruptures.

To begin this exercise, open your *Heart Journey*™ *Journal* to **Individual Heartwork - 360 Quadrant Exercise** A and see the first figure. Notice the female figure is labeled top (T), underneath (U), right (R), and left (L). Imagine this is your body. Notice the figure is divided into six quadrants. Take time to think about the sensations you feel in each quadrant of your own body. Consider whether or not you feel safe or comfortable, mildly unsafe, unsafe or not comfortable, very unsafe, or numb in and about each quadrant of your body. Do not judge what you experience in your felt sense of your body, as what you feel could be related to previous traumas or experiences.

1. If you feel safe, write S or color in green.

2. If you feel mildly unsafe, write MUS or color in yellow.

3. If you feel unsafe or not comfortable, write US or color in orange.

4. If you feel very unsafe, color in red or write VUS.

5. If you feel numb or dissociated from this area, write N or color in blue.

6. Go through this activity for each one of these quadrants.

Take time to gain a felt sense of how each area feels. Track and spend time with your bodily sense. Notice how sensations are being registered in your felt sense and how your brain is perceiving this. If you have a new painful memory that arises as you focus on these quadrants, write it down by that quadrant and go back to Chapter Seven to work it through with Time Reversing Trauma™ Individual Heartwork.

Next, turn to **Individual Heartwork - 360 Quadrant Exercises** B and C in your *Heart Journey™ Journal* and see the figures. We are again going to sense into each quadrant of your body from the left and right side. Take time to think about the sensations you feel in each quadrant of your own body. Consider whether or not you feel safe or comfortable, mildly unsafe, unsafe or not comfortable, very unsafe, or numb in and about each quadrant of your body. Do not judge what you experience in each side (left and right of your body), ask yourself:

Do I feel safe (S; green), mildly unsafe (MUS; yellow), unsafe (US; orange), very unsafe or very vulnerable (VUS; red), or numb (N; blue). Mark each area accordingly, just as you did for figure A.

Last, turn to **Individual Heartwork - 360 Quadrant Exercise D** in your *Heart Journey™ Journal* and see the figure. Imagine yourself looking down upon yourself. Take time to think about the sensations you feel in each quadrant of your own body for this view. Consider whether or not you feel safe or comfortable, mildly unsafe, unsafe or not comfortable, very unsafe, or numb in and about each quadrant of your body. Do not judge what you experience. Again, ask yourself: Do I feel safe (S; green), mildly unsafe (MUS; yellow), unsafe (US; orange), very unsafe or very vulnerable (VUS; red), or numb (N; blue). Mark each area accordingly, just as you did for figure A.

Next you will list every area in which you felt activated (i.e., any area not marked "safe"), and we will pray over each area that you listed, welcoming Jesus into each body area.

## 360 QUADRANT PRAYER ACTIVITY

Complete **Individual Heartwork - 360 Quadrant Exercise** and Activity within your *Heart Journey™ Journal* at this time.

Use this QR code to access audible versions of activities.

## FREEDOM FROM FALSE GUILT

As we wrap up this chapter, this Freedom From False Guilt Activity will allow us to imagine time without guilt or not having that false sense of guilt. God wants you free from all condemnation and accusation (Romans 8:1). This means we must set boundaries in our thought life to keep the false guilt and condemnation out.

Complete **Individual Heartwork - Freedom From False Guilt** within your *Heart Journey*™ *Journal* at this time.

Use this QR code to access audible versions of activities.

## ABUSE

As we end this chapter, we need to talk about a serious issue ... abuse. Abuse is a violation of boundaries and is never acceptable. It can take many forms, including physical, emotional, verbal, sexual, spiritual, financial, and psychological abuse. If you are experiencing abuse, it is important to seek help immediately to ensure your safety and well-being. Abuse can happen in many different types of relationships, including romantic partnerships, family relationships, friendships, and relationships at work or in ministry. It is important to remember that you are not at fault for the abuse you are experiencing, and it is never your responsibility to try to change the abuser's behavior. Abuse is not ever warranted.

It can be difficult to recognize abuse, especially if you have been conditioned to believe that it is normal or that you deserve it. Signs of abuse can include physical injuries, fear of the abuser, isolation from friends and family, changes in behavior or personality, and feeling like you are walking on eggshells around an explosive or controlling abuser.

If you are experiencing abuse, it is important to reach out to a trusted friend or family member, a domestic violence hotline, or a mental health professional for support. They can help you develop a safety plan and provide resources for leaving the abusive situation. Remember that you deserve to be treated with respect and dignity, and that it is never too late to seek help and begin healing from the trauma of abuse.

## BOUNDARIES SHIFT OVER TIME

It is also important to recognize that boundaries can change and evolve over time. As we grow and learn, we may discover that certain boundaries no longer serve us, and we may need to adjust them accordingly. Additionally, different situations may require different boundaries, and it is important to be flexible and adaptive.

## SUPPORT AND GRACE AS YOU GROW

Lastly, as you embark on the journey of growing in a healthy boundaries, it is crucial to prioritize building up your social support network. Often, our struggles with boundaries stem from fears of rejection, hence a strong support system can be invaluable. When we change how we show up in relationships that have been benefitting from our lack of boundaries, we will likely receive negative feedback and possibly rejection. Upping safe social support will act as a buffer for you through the boundary setting hurdles.

Additionally, when we begin setting boundaries, we may find ourselves oscillating between extremes—boundaries that are either too rigid or too flexible. It is important to remember that this is a natural part of the process, and that it is okay to give yourself grace as you navigate through these challenges. Do not hesitate to ask for support and understanding from safe others around you, especially those who truly have your best interest at heart. True friends will stand by you through the ups and downs, providing a steady source of encouragement and strength.

I am so proud of you, Beloved. Be sure to finish your **Individual Heartwork - Chapter Eight Review** and Your *Heart Group Discussion* work with your small group or with a friend. In the upcoming chapter, we delve into the transformative power of forgiveness, encompassing the journey of extending forgiveness to others as well as cultivating self-love. Through this process, we unlock profound healing and liberation, allowing us to embrace the fullness of God's grace and experience the freedom that comes from releasing the burdens of resentment and self-condemnation. So much goodness is ahead!

## LET US PRAY.

*Heavenly Father,*

*Thank You for being with us as we continue on this journey. Working on boundaries challenged us all on so many levels. Help each of us to reestablish healthy boundaries and keep them maintained. And we know that we can only do so by Your strength.*

*Also, Father, thank You for teaching us about the Triangle of Pain. Help us to keep our spiritual eyes open to it and the different enemy attacks that may try to lure us back onto it. Help us to stay strong and to stay off it. Thank You, Father, for continuing to heal these parts of our heart home.*

*In Jesus' name, Amen.*

# *Chapter*

## NINE

### Restoring My Peace

*Then Jesus said to the woman at His feet, "All your sins are forgiven."*
### Luke 7:48 (TPT)

Let me start this chapter by expressing exuberantly, "Well done!" Beloved, you have made so much progress! And, if you are starting to criticize yourself for not doing it perfectly ... stop now and receive the goodness of forward movement!

Now that many of your unmet needs have been met and much of your trauma has been cleared, we can move onto cleaning out the remnants of your heartache through forgiveness. During this part of our journey, we will explore the themes underneath your resentments. We will not just forgive, but will explore the nooks and crannies that still need touches of healing, and allow the light of love and God's goodness into every area of your heart home.

We will work on forgiveness in innovative ways, including using our holy imagination to forgive ourselves at each age and stage of our lives. We will consider where to make amends, from a whole heart, and thereby experience even more healing and closure, realizing that forgiveness does not always mean restoration of trust.

You may wonder why the chapter is titled "Restoring My Peace," yet we are exploring forgiveness of self and others. However, the two concepts are intertwined, and the Bible speaks to this connection. In Matthew 5:9 (LEB), Jesus says, "Blessed are the peacemakers, because they will be called sons of God." The Greek word used here for peacemaker is "eirēnopoios" which means "to endeavor to reconcile persons who have disagreements, making peace." Jesus wants us to make peace with others and with the warring parts of ourselves through forgiveness. Forgiveness is key to your healing and brings us into peace. Giving and receiving forgiveness "makes" deep soul-rich peace.

## UNFORGIVENESS: THE ENEMY'S PLAN

We are now at "U" in our RECONSTRUCTION acronym, which stands for "Unburdening from Resentment." As we continue renovating our heart abodes, why do we need to focus on forgiveness? I cannot tell you how many meetings I have been in where the preacher or teacher asks, "How many of you are struggling with any kind of unforgiveness?" In response, most everyone in the room raises their hand. It is a big problem. Yet, Scripture teaches us that harboring unforgiveness grants an opportunity for the devil to undermine our purpose and bring chaos into our lives.

Throughout this journey, we have witnessed the enemy's relentless attacks on our lives through the painful experiences of trauma, unfulfilled needs, and various forms of abuse. Our hearts yearn for the presence of God alone, desiring to cast out every trace of the enemy's influence where he has managed to establish a foothold in our lives.

*"In your anger do not sin. Do not let the sun go down while you are still angry, and do not give the devil a foothold."*

### Ephesians 4:26-27 (NIV)

Beloved, this Scripture clarifies that allowing unforgiveness and resentment to fester welcomes oppression by the enemy. The word foothold is translated from the Greek word, "topos," which means "a spot, a place, a position, a possibility, passage, or opportunity." Unforgiveness opens the door for the enemy to introduce destruction into your life, and that is something we all desire to avoid.

We are faced with a choice in how we respond to hardships: we can allow bitterness to take root and corrode our hearts, or we can choose forgiveness and embrace The Beautiful Place Prayer™. By surrendering our pain to the Lord, we experience a profound healing that surpasses our expectations. God has the power to transform us as we journey from trauma to forgiveness, and the outcome is beyond anything we could have envisioned. His plans for us are greater than we can ask or imagine.

## FORGIVENESS IS CENTRAL

Moreover, it is essential to recognize that forgiveness is birthed out of the very heart of God's character. If we reflect upon the cross, we find that forgiveness emerges as its central refrain. That pivotal moment in history, which altered the course of humanity and reverberated through the chronicles of time, is fundamentally rooted in the transformative power of forgiveness. The cross stands as a profound testament to God's unwavering commitment to reconcile and restore. It serves as a poignant reminder that forgiveness is not only a divine act but also a foundational principle that permeates every aspect of our existence. The cross, with its resplendent message of forgiveness, encapsulates the extraordinary depth of God's love and the boundless possibilities it holds for our lives.

Forgiveness. Lovely, blessed, lavish, all-encompassing forgiveness. His forgiveness has washed away the most dreadful offenses from sin-soaked humanity, and all we need to do is … receive it? Who is like our God?

> *In Him we have redemption through His blood, the forgiveness of our trespasses, according to the riches of His grace, which He lavished upon us, in all wisdom and insight.*
>
> ### Ephesians 1:7-8 (ESV)

> *Bearing with one another and, if one has a complaint against another, forgiving each other; as the Lord has forgiven you, so you also must forgive.*
>
> ### Colossians 3:13 (ESV)

> *For if you forgive others their trespasses, your Heavenly Father will also forgive you, but if you do not forgive others their trespasses, neither will your Father forgive your trespasses.*
>
> ### Matthew 6:14-15 (ESV)

Beloved, think about everything for which God has forgiven you. Compared to His holiness, we each truly are wretched (Romans 3:23), yet He has given us total and complete forgiveness for every sin we have committed and will commit (Ephesians 1:7)! Consider that every time you go to the Lord, He is uniformly and unwaveringly loving and merciful. He never holds anything against us, when He could, as we behave badly at times. As far as the east is from the west, so far does He remove our transgressions from us (Psalm 103:12, ESV). Yet, He is so good to us, treating us as blameless in His sight.

Yet surprisingly, we hold onto unforgiveness toward others. Oftentimes we ruminate on wrongs done to us as we experience the weight of ache in our hearts. Our anger feels so enticingly justifiable; after all, they wronged us! In Matthew 18, Jesus tells the parable of a king who forgives a servant's enormous debt, but then the same servant refuses to forgive a small debt owed to him by a fellow servant. The king discovers this and scolds the "wicked" servant, reminding him of the mercy he was shown and that he should have extended the same mercy to his fellow servant. Oh, we are so like the servant!

We are not alone, Beloved, as the disciples tussled to surrender to forgiveness as well. In Matthew 18:21-22 (NIV), Peter asked Jesus, "'Lord, how often will my brother sin against me, and I forgive him? As many as seven times?" Jesus said to him, "I do not say to you seven times, but seventy-seven times." Unforgiveness is comparable to drinking poison and expecting the other person to suffer or perish. However, in reality, it is us who suffer and provide an opportunity for the devil to torment us when we hold onto unforgiveness. Thankfully, through the power of Christ, we have the ability to forgive and free ourselves from the toxic grip of resentment.

## FROM BITTER TO LIVING WATER

Forgiveness is a powerful tool that can bring life even after the most painful traumas. It has the power to heal relationships, bring peace to the heart, and transform lives. One of the most inspiring examples of this is the story of the woman at the well in John 4. Let us revisit her story again, this time through the eyes of forgiveness.

You likely recall that the woman at the well was a Samaritan who had been wedded multiple times and was living with a man who was not her husband. Women were not allowed to divorce in her society, so we can suppose she had been rejected repetitively by previous husbands, each break up shattering her heart a bit further. She was an outcast in her community, shunned and excluded to such an extent that she had to fetch water during the hottest hours of the day, possibly to escape the hurtful remarks and judgmental attitudes of the other women in town. However, when she encountered Jesus at the well, her life was transformed. Her previous life died and her new life commenced. He shared with her, "Whoever drinks of the water that I will give him will never be thirsty again. The water that I will give him will become in him a spring of water welling up to eternal life." Jesus did not judge or condemn her, but instead offered her living water and the gift of forgiveness.

Through her transformative encounter with Jesus at the well, the woman discovered the profound power of healing and forgiveness. In leaving behind her painful past, she embraced the gift of forgiveness and chose to extend it to those who had once caused her deep heartache. This remarkable transformation propelled her into a powerful role as a witness for Christ to the very people who had caused her much pain. Her story serves as a powerful testament to the life-altering effects of encountering Christ and embracing the transformative power of forgiveness for self and others.

Furthermore, the woman at the well exemplified extraordinary faith by becoming an early martyr for her beliefs and she is even mentioned alongside the apostles in historical accounts. Her once-painful wounds were transformed into a source of life, symbolizing the abundant grace and redemption available through Christ.

Just as the woman at the well found healing and forgiveness in Christ, we, too, can experience the same transformative power. Regardless of the depth of our wounds or the weight of our pain, God has the ability to turn our past hurts into a river of hope and healing. Through encountering Christ and embracing His forgiveness, we embark on a journey of restoration, becoming vessels of His love, compassion, and grace in the world.

## DEBORAH'S STORY

Deborah experienced the heart-wrenching pain of saying goodbye to her stillborn baby, a tragedy that could have consumed her with bitterness and cause her to raise questions about God's sovereignty.

She could have easily wondered why such a devastating event was allowed to happen. However, Deborah made a remarkable choice: she forgave the harshness of life itself, and placed her trust in the Lord even amidst her grief over the loss of her son, Michael.

Years later, Deborah was given an opportunity to share her journey of healing from child loss with a group of women. As she made her way to the event, a mild hurricane named "Michael" swept through the area, bringing torrents of rain in every direction. It was in that moment, amidst the storm, that the Lord spoke to her, revealing a profound truth. He said, "Because you have entrusted your loss to me and have refused to let bitterness take hold of your heart, I have transformed your pain into a powerful force of life-giving water that flows from within you."

## THE GIFTS OF FORGIVENESS

Forgiveness is an active process that involves letting go of resentment and anger toward those who have wronged us and has many benefits. Forgiveness, or the lack thereof, impacts our mental and physical health, and improves the quality of our relationships with others and the Lord. Forgiveness leads to lower heart rates and blood pressure, resulting in better physical health.[28] Additionally, it can lower symptoms of depression and anxiety, improve overall life satisfaction, and increase empathy and understanding toward others.[29, 30] Moreover, forgiveness brings about a profound sense of liberation, as if a heavy burden has been lifted from our shoulders.

Additionally, forgiveness has a significant impact on our overall countenance. It is fascinating to consider that within each of us exists an elder version of ourselves, longing for a life characterized by peace, joy, and forgiveness. As we journey through life, our facial appearance becomes a reflection of the choices we make. Our repeated choices are etched on our faces, appearing as wrinkles that convey whether our lives have been illuminated by love and joy or clouded by bitterness and resentment. Don't you aspire to radiate with light and exude joy? That elder version of yourself is urging you to make wise choices, recognizing that one day, it will be you looking back and yearning for a life marked by forgiveness. So, why not start today? Embrace forgiveness, knowing that it will draw you closer to the light and joy you deeply desire.

Forgiveness also impacts our spiritual clarity. Mark 11:25 (NIV) tells us, "When you stand praying, if you hold anything against anyone, forgive them, so that your Father in heaven may forgive you your sins." Even though we are forgiven through Jesus Christ, forgiveness is linked to the flow of God's blessings in our lives. I have heard stories of people who really tried to obey, but harbored bitterness and judgement; and then of other people who had messy Christian lives, but were very forgiving. Typically, the forgiving people enjoyed God's blessings more than the judgmental people, because judgment and unforgiveness are not in God's heart for us.

## FEAR AND RESENTMENT

As we embark on the journey of working through our unforgiveness and resentments, we will inevitably encounter various threads and strands of fear woven into the fabric of our lives. The Lord, in His loving kindness, desires to bring healing to these areas of fear. It is worth noting that resentment often becomes intertwined with fear, alongside a sense of self-preservation rooted in selfishness.

Throughout the Bible, we can find insightful passages that illuminate the connection between fear and resentment. In Psalm 37:8 (NIV), it says, "Refrain from anger and turn from wrath; do not fret—it leads only to evil." This verse highlights how dwelling in anger and harboring resentment can lead to a spiraling path that encompasses fear and ultimately leads to harmful actions and attitudes.

Furthermore, in 1 John 4:18 (NIV), we are reminded that "There is no fear in love. But perfect love drives out fear because fear has to do with punishment. The one who fears is not made perfect in love." This verse emphasizes the contrast between fear and love, indicating that fear finds its roots in a sense of punishment and is antithetical to the perfect love that comes from God.

As we let go of resentment and embrace forgiveness, we can break free from the grip of fear and selfish self-preservation. In doing so, we open ourselves up to a journey of healing and growth, guided by God's perfect love.

## IDENTIFYING RESENTMENTS

Resentment is a series of thoughts and attitudes that result in an intricate emotion. It is an internal experience characterized by deep-seated thoughts and feelings of bitterness, anger, or indignation directed toward a person or a situation perceived as causing harm, offense, or injustice. It often arises when we feel wronged, betrayed, triggered, or mistreated in some way.

Internally, resentment can manifest as a heavy weight on the heart and a persistent sense of discontentment or displeasure. It may consume our thoughts and emotions, causing us to replay the perceived wrongdoing repeatedly in our minds. Resentment can generate a sense of injustice, fueling a desire for vindication or retribution.

The experience of resentment may involve a mix of negative emotions such as anger, frustration, hurt, and disappointment. It can lead to a sense of being emotionally drained, as it takes a significant toll on our mental and emotional well-being. In some cases, resentment may also contribute to feelings of powerlessness or victimhood, as it keeps us locked in a cycle of negativity and prevents us from moving forward.

In the Bible, we are reminded to, "Get rid of all bitterness, rage and anger, brawling and slander, along with every form of malice. Be kind and compassionate to one another, forgiving each other, just as in Christ God forgave you" (Ephesians 4:31-32, NIV).

To identify resentments, it is essential to reflect on past experiences and relationships. This can include situations where our needs were not met or when we felt wronged or mistreated by someone. You will look through your *Heart Journey*™ *Journal* Chapter Five timelines and identify those who have caused trauma or unmet needs. You will also sit before the Lord and ask Him who else needs to be added to your list. "God" and "life in general" should also be on your list.

Now it is time to reopen your *Heart Journey*™ *Journal* and complete the exercise in Chapter Nine, **Individual Heartwork - Identifying Resentments**. We will use this list as we continue our Unburdening from Resentment™: Others work.

## UNBURDENING FROM RESENTMENT™: OTHERS

The **Individual Heartwork - Unburdening from Resentment**™ involves working through resentments toward others, God, and life. Cleaning the heart home from all debris, including dust under the appliances that is not easily seen, is crucial as Jesus asks us to clean our inner heart chambers (Mathew 5:8; Matthew 23:25-26; Proverbs 4:23). In this chapter, we will wash our hearts clean from resentment using a chart with four columns - "The Person I Resent," "Why I Resent That Person," "What is Threatened?" and "My Part." This activity combines Scripture, Forgiveness Theory, and 12-step tools and is effective in transforming individuals to become all God made them to be. It promotes forgiveness and healing, leading to emotional, mental, and spiritual well-being.

## DEBORAH'S STORY

When Deborah first sat down to do the Unburdening from Resentment™ Heartwork activity, she was surprised to discover how many resentments she had buried deep within her heart. She took the time for a thorough exploration, particularly regarding her relationship with her mother, Jeanne. Deborah's mother had frequently kicked her out of their family home in a drunken rage and refused to let her back in. As a child, Deborah had to wait in the dark corner of the apartment complex in her pajamas until her mother had passed out, and her younger brother would then sneak her back in. These experiences threatened Deborah's basic needs for survival and belonging, and they had long-lasting effects on her emotional and physical sense of safety, her sense of love and belonging, and her self-esteem.

As she worked through the exercise, Deborah took a hard look at her own role in the situation. She realized that her fear of rejection and abandonment, which had taken root in her close relationships and especially with her spouse, was her part in perpetuating the cycle of resentment. She owned up to this fear and forgave herself, her mother, and everyone else on her resentment list.

Through the process of forgiving herself and others, Deborah experienced a profound shift in her heart. She did not feel the change immediately, but it came soon after. She also shared her Unburdening from Resentment™ Heartwork with a trusted friend and prayed with them for the healing of her heart. This proved to be a very liberating experience.

Now complete your **Individual Heartwork - Unburdening from Resentment™: Others.**

Remember, forgiveness is not a feeling. It becomes a feeling over time, but it starts out as a choice. As you continue cleaning the deep crevices of your heart home, all that unwanted grime and mildew that have built up over the years, choose to forgive each one of these people.

Now we will work on forgiving yourself over time.

# UNBURDENING FROM RESENTMENT™ - SELF AT EVERY AGE

My friend, often we carry in our heart the oppressive weight of self-criticism and judgments we have exercised against ourselves for decades. Most of us have nitpicked and even hated elements of ourselves throughout the various stages of our lives. This has had a cumulative and detrimental impact on our sense of self. Like a brilliant piece of art that has been vandalized, our self-image over time has been mangled and tinted with the jagged blades of shame and blame. These burdens impact our relationships, self-esteem, confidence, and overall well-being. It is time to forgive ourselves, and embrace love and acceptance.

Imagine if you had to bear the burden of carrying a small rock for every self-judgment you have held throughout your life. Pause for a moment and reflect on the weight of those rocks accumulated over time. How heavy would your load be? Dear friend, even the smallest self-hatreds and self-condemnation are silently imposing immense weight upon you. It is time to give this weight to Jesus.

To begin this journey of self-acceptance and forgiveness, we will reflect on the different periods of our lives and the judgments we placed upon ourselves during those times. Looking at old photographs of ourselves at various stages of life can help us remember how we viewed ourselves. Did we judge ourselves harshly, feeling inadequate, not smart enough, or lacking in attractiveness? We want to look at how we felt about ourselves across three domains: who we were (our personality), what we did (our choices), and our physical appearance. Physical appearance often becomes an area of intense self-criticism, particularly for women, so it is crucial to address body- and beauty-shaming as well.

For instance, during the ages of zero to five, did you feel loved, safe, and protected, or did you experience feelings of neglect, loneliness, or abandonment? What beliefs did you hold about yourself during those formative years? We will continue this reflection for ages six through ten, eleven through fourteen, fifteen through eighteen, and to our current age.

Here, we are reminded of the Scriptures that guide us toward self-acceptance, forgiveness, and love. One such passage is found in Mark 12:30-31 (NIV), where Jesus teaches us the greatest commandment: "Love the Lord your God with all your heart and with all your soul and with all your mind and with all your strength. The second is this: 'Love your neighbor as yourself.' There is no commandment greater than these." This Scripture challenges us to choose to love God more than our self-criticisms, rejections, and unforgiveness. It invites us to shift our focus from dwelling on our flaws and past mistakes to embracing God's love and forgiveness.

The challenge before us is willingness to surrender our past self-rejections to God. We must choose to trust His work on the cross rather than be willful about holding onto self-rejection. Let us revisit 1 John 4:18 (NIV), which says, "There is no fear in love. But perfect love drives out fear because fear has to do with punishment. The one who fears is not made perfect in love." It is time to allow God's perfect love to replace our self-criticism and self-shaming. Only then will we experience the freedom that comes from embracing our true identity as beloved children of God.

We can draw upon the parable of the lost coin from Luke 15:8-10. In this parable, a woman diligently searches for a lost coin, rejoicing when she finds it. In a similar way, Jesus seeks the lost parts of our hearts that are hidden in self-rejection and shame. He desires to bring every part of us into His love and acceptance at every age and stage.

To truly abide in the Lord and experience oneness with Him, we must align our hearts and minds with His. This alignment starts with accepting, loving, and forgiving ourselves at every moment of our history. It is through this process that we can fully agree with our Maker and embrace the profound truth that "God is love" (1 John 4:8, ESV). In order to agree with God, we must let go of self-contempt and self-condemnation. We must recognize that God's love extends to every moment of our lives, even the ones we deem unworthy or tainted by mistakes. His love is unconditional and boundless, reaching into the depths of our shame to heal and make us whole.

The blood of Jesus, shed on the cross, has the power to reach every nook and cranny of our past, present, and future. It is through His sacrifice that we find redemption, forgiveness, and restoration. When we accept, love, and forgive ourselves, we allow His transformative love to permeate every aspect of our being. God's forgiveness is limitless.

Loving ourselves means embracing our uniqueness, embracing our strengths and weaknesses, and embracing the journey we are on. It means treating ourselves with compassion, grace, and kindness, just as God treats us. When we love ourselves, we open ourselves up to experiencing the depths of God's love for us and can extend that love to others and back to Him. We are like a soda bottle floating in the ocean of God's love and grace. There is more than enough to fill us.

In Luke chapter seven, we meet the woman who washed Jesus' feet with her hair and tears after experiencing His grace and forgiveness. Upon realizing the depths of her own forgiveness and acceptance, she could not contain her joy and chose to make a bold gesture in front of those who would judge her. With tears streaming down her face, she washed Jesus' feet with her hair and anointed them with expensive perfume. Her gratitude and love overflowed, prompting her to offer her most valuable possessions as a sign of her devotion.

Likewise, when we grasp the magnitude of God's love and forgiveness in our own lives, we are no longer defined by our past mistakes or burdened by guilt and shame. We are set free to live our lives marked by joy, gratitude, and love.

When we choose to forgive ourselves and embrace love and acceptance across all ages, we learn to love even the most vulnerable parts of ourselves. We can release the heavy burden of self-judgment and criticism, freeing ourselves to live a life of freedom, self-compassion, and acceptance.

However, there is an insidious force that seeks to keep us trapped in self-unforgiveness, preventing us from fully embracing God's love and forgiveness. The enemy, in his cunning ways, uses our imperfections, past mistakes, regrets, and failures as weapons to attack our self-worth and keep us stuck in a cycle of self-condemnation.

But I urge you, my dear friend, do not give in to the enemy's schemes. Rise up with courage and determination to break free from the chains of self-unforgiveness. Stand firm in the truth of God's Word and His limitless grace. The blood of Jesus, shed on the cross, has the power to cleanse and redeem every aspect of your life, including your self-inflicted wounds.

Let us delve into Deborah's story, where she carried the deep wounds of childhood rejection. Abandoned by both her parents and left homeless at seventeen, Deborah struggled to see her own worthiness of love. Through her *Heart Journey*™, Jesus unveiled the truth of her inherent lovability. He revealed that she was fearfully and wonderfully made, deserving of acceptance and love. Deborah embarked on a path of forgiveness, starting with her parents and moving onto herself. As she gradually learned to nurture her inner child with compassion and embraced the love extended by Jesus, a remarkable transformation unfolded. Shedding self-criticism and judgment, Deborah wholeheartedly embraced the love and acceptance offered by Jesus, allowing her inherent lovability to blossom, little by little. This newfound self-image radiated through her relationships, bringing healing and connection.

Like Deborah, you are not defined by your past. You are not defined by your mistakes. You are not defined by your shortcomings. You are not defined by the world's standards. Your worth and belonging are found in Christ, Who has loved you, chosen you, forgiven you and set you free. The enemy may try to remind you of your failures, but you have the authority to declare that you are forgiven, loved, and accepted by God.

I charge you now, my friend, to release yourself from the grip of self-unforgiveness and self-criticism. Let go of the self-condemnation that weighs you down and embrace the freedom that comes from accepting God's forgiveness. Allow His love to wash over you, cleansing you from the inside out. It is time, Beloved, it has long been time. Now, reopen your *Heart Journey™ Journal* and complete the exercise in Chapter Nine, **Individual Heartwork - Unburdening from Resentment™: Self at Every Age** and then complete the **Forgiving Myself Activity**.

Use this QR code to access audible versions of activities.

## MAKING AMENDS

Now we will continue to get free from burdens of your past by making amends. Look through your resentment list at the "My Part" section from your **Individual Heartwork - Unburdening from Resentment™: Others**, and consider to whom you need to make amends. It is likely you will be on this list as well. Yes, you need to make amends to yourself! In addition, it is time to make amends to those you have harmed.

Sometimes, we make amends through paying back what is owed, other times we change our behavior, and many times we also apologize. We own our part and make amends even if we never receive a desired apology or amends from the other. Jesus commanded, "Love your enemies and pray for those who persecute you, that you may be children of your Father in heaven. He causes His sun to rise on the evil and the good, and sends rain on the righteous and the unrighteous. If you love those who love you, what reward will you get? Are not even the tax collectors doing that?" (Matthew 5:44-46, NIV). Making amends not only restores our relationships but also brings healing to our hearts and pleases the Lord. As we delve into the process of making amends, we discover it has a profound impact on our inner being and our connection with God.

In Matthew 5:23-24 (ESV), Jesus teaches us about the importance of making things right, "So if you are offering your gift at the altar and there remember that your brother has something against you, leave your gift there before the altar and go. First, be reconciled to your brother, and then come and offer your gift." This passage reminds us that we must stop looking at our sister's or brother's fault, and take care of what is on our side of the street in the matter. It emphasizes the significance of making amends and seeking reconciliation as a priority before presenting our offerings to the Lord.

In Luke 19:1-10 (ESV), the story of Zacchaeus beautifully illustrates the profound healing power of making amends. Zacchaeus said to the Lord, "Behold, Lord, the half of my goods I give to the poor. And if I have defrauded anyone of anything, I restore it fourfold." Then Jesus replied to him, "Today salvation has come to this house, since he also is a son of Abraham. For the Son of Man came to seek and to save the lost."

Beloved, when we make amends, the lost parts of our hearts experience the deep wells of restoration. Making amends is part of our healing as we participate with Jesus in reversing the ripple effects of sin. Moreover, the burdens of conscious are lifted, allowing our hearts to swim in seas of peace and completeness.

## DEBORAH'S STORY

Let us look at Deborah's life as an example of how God leads the amends process. Deborah and her younger brother decided to visit their grandparents' house, which brought them to the area where they lived as children. Led by the Lord's prompting, they felt compelled to reconnect with their old neighbors, guided by God's direction to visit a specific house. After twenty years of no contact, they dropped in to greet them. Surprisingly, the oldest daughter, who had recently expressed guilt for her past mistreatment of Deborah to her mother, had shared her desire to apologize. And just days later, Deborah appeared at their doorstep, having not seen each other for decades. After being bullied by the daughter, Deborah had harassed the family via prank calls for several years as a tween. Deborah took the opportunity to apologize. What followed was a beautiful time of reconciliation, where Deborah discovered that the parents of the girl who bullied her had been praying for Deborah's salvation throughout the years. They were overjoyed to learn that Deborah was now following Jesus. This remarkable encounter showcased God's perfect timing and orchestrating of amends. It was undeniably led by Him, as He took care of Deborah's journey of making amends. Be encouraged that God will do the same for you, leading you in your own amends process. Your part is to obey.

Now, reopen your *Heart Journey*™ *Journal* and complete the exercise in Chapter Nine, **Individual Heartwork - Making Amends.**

## THREE TYPES OF FORGIVENESS

As we go through the process of making amends, it is important to know there are three types of forgiveness as it is related to reconciliation. Reconciliation means restoring a broken relationship and working toward healing and rebuilding trust. It involves both parties actively participating in the process and addressing the issues that caused the rift. Reconciliation requires sincere repentance, genuine change, and a willingness to make amends. It is a mutual effort that aims to establish a healthy and respectful connection, guided by open communication, understanding, and forgiveness. However, it is essential to prioritize safety and well-being in the process, especially in cases of abuse or harmful behavior, where reconciliation may not be possible or advisable.

First, we will consider **forgiveness with no reconciliation**. Here, we choose to forgive, but there can be no reconciliation in the relationship. This occurs when: the person will not reconcile with us even though we want to reconcile; the person has passed; or, having a relationship with that person puts us, our children, or something or someone important to us in any type of danger. For example, if one's grandfather is a known pedophile and hurt family members, we can forgive him, but we will not allow him near our children. Moreover, we should report him to the authorities to prevent more children from being harmed.

There is also **forgiveness with partial reconciliation**. In this case, we choose to forgive the person and pray for God's blessings upon them, but due to their lack of repentance for the harm they caused, or due to the extent of trust broken, only a partial restoration of the relationship is appropriate. While forgiveness is extended freely, trust needs to be earned. Without genuine repentance, it is only possible to allow them into our lives to a limited extent.

For example, let us say you have a deep bond with your best friend, but she made a serious attempt to seduce your husband. Even if she wholeheartedly repents, it is unlikely you will ever fully trust her as you did before. The betrayal and display of poor character have deeply impacted the trust between you. While you may still interact pleasantly, you must establish healthy boundaries and protect your family by not granting her access to loved ones. In another example, Deborah forgave her ex-husband who left her for another woman. At the same time, trust was deeply broken and unless he showed the fruits of long-term repentance, she would not reconcile the marriage.

The third type is **forgiveness with full reconciliation** which can be challenging, but rewarding. As daughters of the King, we must remain open to the possibility of complete restoration, particularly when the person shows genuine repentance and there are no safety concerns involved. As believers, we recognize that God is a God of reconciliation, and He desires reconciliation in many cases. 2 Corinthians 5:18 (NIV) tells us, "All this is from God, who reconciled us to Himself through Christ and gave us the ministry of reconciliation." God's work of reconciliation through Jesus Christ extends to us, and we are called to reflect His love and grace by pursuing reconciliation with others.

## DEBORAH'S STORY

An inspiring example of forgiveness with reconciliation can be found in Deborah's personal journey. Deborah and her brother had a strained relationship for many years due to his reckless lifestyle and struggles with substance abuse. Witnessing her brother's repeated brushes with death and encounters with the law, Deborah felt a growing detachment from him, as she believed he could not consistently be available in the relationship. While she still loved and forgave him for his off-and-on unavailability, she felt the need to create some emotional distance to protect her own heart from the tumultuous ups and downs of his life.

However, over time, Deborah's brother began to make positive changes and embraced a more stable and spiritual path. His transformation and the prompting of the Holy Spirit sparked a realization within Deborah that she should not let fear of potential disappointments hold her back from cultivating a deeper connection with him. She confronted her fears head-on and made a conscious decision to pursue a more profound and authentic relationship with her brother. By taking this brave step toward reconciliation, Deborah allowed herself to be vulnerable and open to the possibilities of healing and growth.

As we can see through Deborah's story, it takes courage, patience, and a willingness to step beyond our fears to rebuild fractured relationships. But the rewards of reconnecting on a deeper level and experiencing the transformative power of love and forgiveness are immeasurable. Where He leads, we must follow.

Seeking guidance from licensed professionals or informed spiritual mentors can be essential when navigating the complexities of reconciliation. They can provide valuable insights and perspectives to help you make informed decisions. However, it is crucial to prioritize safety above all else. Remember, your safety and the well-being of those around you are of utmost importance. Trust your instincts and listen to the Holy Spirit's voice when making decisions about reconciliation.

## STICKY RESENTMENTS

At times, despite our decision to forgive, we may find our resentments still cling to us, causing inner turmoil. As you progress in your *Heart Journey*™ and engage in the process of making amends, you might come across Sticky Resentments. These are resentments that persist and hold us back from experiencing true freedom and peace.

To find relief from these Sticky Resentments, one powerful practice is to pray for those whom we resent. This act of prayer opens our hearts and allows us to surrender to the love of the Father. Scripture reminds us of the transformative power of praying for our enemies and those who have wronged us. In Matthew 5:44 (NIV), Jesus instructs us to "love your enemies and pray for those who persecute you." We are called to sincerely pray for the well-being and blessings we would like most for ourselves for these people. Through prayer, we not only get relief from resentment and healing, but also surrender to being filled with divine love and grace.

## DEBORAH'S STORY

Despite diligently completing her Heartwork, Deborah found herself resenting a particular woman who had caused significant turmoil within her family. Forgiving this person proved to be a challenging task for Deborah, and she experienced the resentment as burdensome and obsessive. Deborah used the *Heart Journey*™ Sticky Resentments tool and prayed for this woman. Twice a day, she fervently prayed for this woman, asking for the same blessings she desired for herself.

As Deborah committed herself to this practice, she experienced a remarkable transformation within herself. The weight of resentment gradually lifted, and a profound sense of mental and emotional freedom enveloped her. It was a beautiful and liberating experience. But what amazed her even more was witnessing the tangible changes unfolding in the life of the woman she prayed for.

Unexpectedly, the woman began to undergo a transformation. She started changing and growing in lovely ways that Deborah never anticipated. Deborah realized that while she had initially prayed to break free from resentment, she had not anticipated the positive impact it would have on the other person's life. She realized that by surrendering her resentment and sincerely praying for the well-being of others, she had played a part in facilitating their transformation.

Now, reopen your *Heart Journey*™ *Journal* and complete the exercise in Chapter Nine, **Individual Heartwork - Sticky Resentments.**

## EMPTY CHAIR: CHRISTIAN VERSION

The Empty Chair Christian Version offers a great way to work through resentment in a relationship, especially when it may not be possible to see the person, or if you are still struggling with the situation. We have already been introduced to this tool in previous chapters. Feel free to use this tool with Sticky Resentments. Imagine and practice pouring out your heart to the person you resent, telling them all you want them to hear while Jesus strengthens and supports you. Then tell them what they did was wrong, but you forgive them based on the finished work of Jesus on the cross.

## A GARDEN WITHOUT WEEDS

Beloved, we now wrap up this chapter on forgiveness and prepare to participate more deeply in all things being restored in Chapter Ten. Before moving on, take time to complete your **Individual Heartwork and Heart Group Discussion** work in your journal.

And regarding our forgiveness work, let us remember that forgiveness is a continual choice of surrendering to the Lord. As emphasized in Colossians 3:13, forgiveness is not a one-time event, but an ongoing process rooted in God's forgiveness toward us. This continuous act of forgiveness is supported by psychological research, which highlights its positive influence on mental health outcomes and overall life satisfaction.

*Bear with each other and forgive one another if any of you has a grievance against someone. Forgive as the Lord forgave you.*

### Colossians 3:13 (NIV)

Moreover, it is crucial to recognize that forgiveness necessitates daily maintenance, akin to tending to a garden. Just as we diligently remove weeds to protect the fruitfulness of a garden, we must actively fence out the enemy of resentment from our lives. This means regularly examining our hearts, seeking the Lord's guidance, and letting go of bitterness and the desire for revenge. By intentionally nurturing forgiveness and surrendering to the Lord, we create a space for healing, restoration, and the transformative power of His grace and love to flourish within us. Now we move on to deeper pools of restoration and living the higher life in Him.

*As the heavens are higher than the earth, so are My ways higher than your ways and My thoughts than your thoughts.*

Isaiah 55:9 (NIV)

## LET US PRAY.

*Heavenly Father,*

*I am beginning to feel so free ... free from resentments, unforgiveness, and so many issues that have weighed heavy on my heart for far too long. Thank You for being with us as we continue on this journey. Please continue to show us areas that may still need renovation. We want to heal fully, and know that can only happen through Your loving guidance. Thank You, Father, for continuing to heal these parts of our heart home.*

*In Jesus' name, Amen.*

# *Chapter*

## TEN

### Restoring My Lost Opportunities

*Therefore, if anyone is in Christ, the new creation has come:*
*The old has gone, the new is here!*
**2 Corinthians 5:17 (NIV)**

By now, you may find yourself embracing the radiant transformation of your heart. As we have diligently worked on restoring and renovating your heart home, it is time to shift our focus toward filling it with the abundant goodness of God. We are entering a phase of decoration and beautification, where we will adorn the newly renovated spaces with tools which will help you live more confidently and jubilantly. Through this process, we will explore the myriad of ways to welcome and embrace greater restoration, delight, enjoyment, and self-discipline into our lives. We will also participate with the Lord in Reclaiming Lost Opportunities from our pasts, and acquire skills that enhance our enjoyment of life.

In our RECONSTRUCTION acronym, we are going to focus on "C," which stands for "Cede to a New Way of Living." Cede means to yield. As you reflect on your journey thus far, you may have encountered moments when it felt overwhelming to surrender and yield to the Lord. However, through numerous transformative encounters with Jesus, we begin to experience a deepening intimacy and connection with Him. These encounters soften our hearts and draw us closer to Him, allowing us to approach Him with renewed trust and openness. Although we are laying down our sinful nature, we are not giving up our true selves. We are yielding to our true selves, made to serve God in gratitude and full of gladness. We are enfolding ourselves into Him to be enraptured in daily encounters with Him. In our journey, we are discovering the power of fixing our gaze upon Jesus and entrusting Him with the challenges and problems of this world.

## CEDE TO ACCEPTANCE

First, we embrace ceding to acceptance. Have you heard the Serenity Prayer before? "God, grant me the serenity to accept the things I cannot change, the courage to change the things I can, and the wisdom to know the difference." This powerful prayer offers much wisdom, encouraging us to accept that which we cannot change, which is usually other people, places, and things. But, in this prayer, we are "owning" what we can change, which is ourselves. As a gift, this prayer reminds us that we are not powerless. We have ourselves, and we have the Lord. Often, we focus on trying to change others, which is futile, rather than changing the one person we can— us. Oh, what glorious freedom we have! We can accept others, while accomplishing all we need to through Him who gives us strength (Philippians 4:13). We have a spirit of power, love, and sound mind (2 Timothy 1:7)!

## THE TIM PRINCIPLE

I appreciate what I refer to as "The Tim Principle," named after my husband, Tim. This principle consists of three parts. First, it involves having an attitude of allowing others to make their own choices. Recognizing and respecting their right to make decisions is essential. Secondly, it means refraining from passing judgment. While we can still adhere to biblical principles and discern what is right and wrong, we should avoid criticism, judgment, disdain, and a critical spirit, as highlighted in Matthew 7:1-5. Lastly, it entails making a deliberate choice about our own involvement. Just because someone is engaged in something and we choose not to judge it, does not mean we automatically participate. We should exercise discernment and refrain from enabling behaviors that go against our values.

Now, let us embark on our Heartwork, applying the wisdom of the Serenity Prayer and the principles of The Tim Principle™ to cede to acceptance. Reopen your *Heart Journey™ Journal* and complete the exercise in Chapter Ten **Individual Heartwork - Cede to Acceptance.**

## CEDE TO GRATITUDE

Gratitude, although it may seem cliché, holds incredible power. I often witness its transformative effects when working with clients. One way to demonstrate this power is by inviting them to create a list of things they are grateful for, even if they appear simple or fundamental, such as the ability to see, hear, or enjoy good health. It is remarkable how their mood can instantly shift through this practice.

Now, let us explore a fresh perspective on reflecting upon the past. Take a moment to consider the resources that sustained you during difficult times. Have you ever paused to contemplate that? Your past traumas, despite their challenges, have endowed you with unique strengths and abilities. Our aim is to uncover and utilize these gifts!

What inner and external resources aided you in navigating through those trying moments?

## DEBORAH'S STORY

As Deborah reflected on her past in her Heartwork, she recognized the ways her unwavering determination and tenacity enabled her to overcome challenges. She also appreciated certain coping strategies that were not initially healthy for her, such as addictive behaviors, which served as survival mechanisms during horrific periods of her life. However, she is grateful that she has been able to let go of those detrimental habits. While acknowledging the need for repentance, she can even find gratitude in the fact that they played a role in her survival.

Moreover, Deborah's traumas have gifted her with a profound sense of empathy for others, a valuable attribute that arose from her own experiences. Additionally, after years of needing to be attuned to danger signals for violence in her parents, she has developed a remarkable ability to read a room, intuitively sensing the dynamics and atmosphere in various situations. Now it is your turn to find the superpowers you developed through your traumas and trials.

Open your *Heart Journey*™ *Journal* in Chapter Ten to **Individual Heartwork - Cede to Gratitude.**

## CEDE TO SPIRITUAL DISCIPLINE

Beloved, we have diligently cleared away significant rubble from your trauma on this transformative journey, attending to the places where your unmet needs once resided. As a result, the practice of spiritual disciplines can become more firmly established in your life. Embracing discipline entails cultivating healthy habits in the Lord, even when our emotions may not align with our intentions. We are called to walk by faith and not be governed solely by our feelings. The time has come for you to surrender to the pursuit of spiritual disciplines, thereby enabling your spiritual growth to unfold fully in accordance with the divine plan for your life. The subsequent overview provides a glimpse into a few key spiritual disciplines from our rich Christian heritage that will help you cede to more of Him in your life.[31] We have removed trauma, now we must fill up with Him.

**The Discipline of Prayer.** The daily, hourly, and even continuous practice of prayer is essential for maintaining a deep connection with our Heavenly Father. In order to have a relationship with anyone, we must communicate with them and receive their communications. Our relationship with the Lord is no different. Within the realm of prayer, there exist various forms and approaches, but in this context, we focus on the significance of praying for God's kingdom to come and His will to be done (Matthew 6:10). We need not fear continuously seeking His intervention in our lives and in the lives of our loved ones.

Prayer is a dynamic dialogue between us and God, where we not only express our hearts, but also listen attentively to His response. Moreover, He answers our prayers, not always in the way we request, but always in the affirmative when we pray His will. "Therefore, I tell you, whatever you ask in prayer, believe that you have received it, and it will be yours" (Mark 11:24, ESV). Therefore, we pray in faith, and attempt to pray along the lines of His revealed will.

In following the example of our friend Deborah, we can take a moment to reflect on our areas of responsibility and influence. Deborah prayerfully intercedes for her team at work, her children, her family, and the small group she and her husband lead. This approach provides a helpful framework for constructing a prayer list. Similarly, I adopt a similar practice by offering prayers for every aspect of my life for which I hold responsibility.

Moreover, I engage in heartfelt conversations with God, often asking, "Father, what are Your thoughts on this?" Sometimes, while reading His word, I pose questions like, "Jesus, why did You do that?" and remarkably, He responds. He wants us to talk with Him about everything. He says, "no longer do I call you servants, for the servant does not know what his master is doing; but I have called you friends, for all that I have heard from My Father I have made known to you" (John 15:15, ESV). His heart wishes to share His whole self with us as we do the same with Him.

Listening is an invaluable part of prayer, and we can be deeply grateful for the wisdom imparted through James 1:5 (NIV), which teaches, "If any of you lacks wisdom, you should ask God, who gives generously to all without finding fault, and it will be given to you." James 1:6 (NIV) further emphasizes the importance of unwavering faith, admonishing us not to doubt: "But when you ask, you must believe and not doubt, because the one who doubts is like a wave of the sea, blown and tossed by the wind." Here, we see He will talk to us; we just need to inquire of Him.

By integrating prayer and practicing Pneumaception™, the art of listening to the Holy Spirit, into our day-to-day rhythms, we create space for a deeper connection with God. In the midst of life's uncertainties, these intentional practices become vital tools for seeking God's wisdom and guidance. His voice is life for our souls. Furthermore, our voice is life to Him, "My dove in the clefts of the rock, in the hiding places on the mountainside, show me your face, let me hear your voice; for your voice is sweet, and your face is lovely." (Song of Solomon 2:14, NIV). Your voice is sweet and lovely to Him.

**The Discipline of Reading the Word.** Another vital spiritual discipline is the intentional regular reading of God's Word, which can be approached in various ways: conducting topical studies, delving into word studies, reading or listening through entire books, or exploring the lives of biblical characters. If you have not delved into the Bible extensively and regularly, I highly recommend starting with the New Testament, particularly the gospels. They beautifully portray Jesus and showcase His profound love for humanity while teaching us how to live in Him.

When we engage in the sacred act of reading God's Word, we discover that it reads us in return. As the Scriptures proclaim, "For the word of God is living and active, sharper than any two-edged sword, piercing to the division of soul and of spirit, of joints and of marrow, and discerning the thoughts and intentions of the heart" (Hebrews 4:12, ESV). Scripture possesses the remarkable ability to penetrate the depths of our being, unveiling the true state of our souls.

During my personal encounters with the Scriptures, I have experienced profound moments when God intentionally illuminates a particular passage, speaking directly to the depths of my heart. It is as if He is whispering a personal message from His heart to mine, revealing His divine insight, comfort, and guidance. These divine highlights within the pages of the Bible serve as intimate connections between the Creator and the created, a sacred exchange that transforms our lives from the inside out.

Deborah, in her personal journey with Jesus, testifies that she has never found Him to be impatient or harsh. Even when He challenges her to make changes or calls her to repentance, His approach is always grace-filled and uplifting, with a constant invitation to rise higher. My own experience mirrors this truth, as I have discovered Jesus to be consistently tender and kindhearted (Matthew 11:28-30). As we spend time immersed in the Scriptures, we begin to discern the distinct voices speaking to us—the voice of our own desires, the voice of the enemy, and the voice of the Holy Spirit. It becomes evident that the voice of the Holy Spirit continually calls us to greater heights, providing encouragement, truth, and grace.

When engaging in the study of God's Word, it is crucial to maintain a balance between truth and grace. Personally, I find it helpful to regularly ask myself, "Am I leaning too heavily toward perceiving God as strict and demanding?" If the answer is yes, it indicates a need to delve deeper into the concepts of grace, God's love, and acceptance. Similarly, if I find myself excessively focused on God's lavish love while lacking discipline in my own life, it signals the necessity of studying the principles of discipline. Thus, it is vital to maintain a well-rounded diet of God's Word, incorporating various themes and aspects, just as a balanced physical diet consists of multiple food groups.

**The Discipline of Waiting on the Lord.** Another spiritual discipline that holds tremendous value is the practice of waiting on the Lord, akin to Mary sitting at the feet of Jesus. It brings to mind those beautiful moments when we are deeply in love with someone, and words become secondary as we simply cherish being in their presence. Similarly, we can find solace and unity with our Heavenly Father by drawing near to Him, resting at His feet, and experiencing the warm and deeply comforting richness of fellowship.

When I intentionally seek to be in His embrace via **The Cuddling Tool**™, I feel the warmth and tenderness of His loving Spirit enveloping me. It is during these precious times that He often speaks directly to my heart, revealing His truths, imparting wisdom, and pouring His love into my being. There is an undeniable increase in the presence of the Holy Spirit as I humbly position myself before Him, and I am reluctant to leave that sacred space.

Isaiah 55:1-3 (AMP) beautifully captures the heart of God's invitation: "Everyone who thirsts, come to the waters; And you who have no money come, buy grain and eat. Come, buy wine and milk without money and without cost (simply accept the gift from God). Why do you spend your money for that which is not bread, and your earnings for what does not satisfy? Listen carefully to Me, and eat what is good, and let your soul delight in abundance. Incline your ear (to listen) and come to Me; Hear, so that your soul may live. And I will make an everlasting covenant with you, according to the faithful mercies (promised and) shown to David." This powerful Scripture underscores God's deep longing for our intimate presence, His desire to commune with us and unveil the wonders of His heart.

**The Discipline of Worship and Praise.** The discipline of worship and praise holds a remarkable power, allowing us to align ourselves with our true purpose as creations designed to glorify and praise our Heavenly Father. When we lift up the name of Jesus with adoration and reverence, something extraordinary happens. His magnetic presence draws all people and every part of our hearts closer to Him. In the act of worship, we are blessed with a profound sense of unity, not only with our Creator but also with one another.

The Scriptures offer affirmations of the transformative impact of heartfelt worship and praise. Isaiah 26:3 (ESV) beautifully assures us, "You keep Him in perfect peace whose mind is stayed on you because He trusts in you." As we fix our minds on the Lord, immersing ourselves in worship, we find ourselves dwelling in the mind of Christ. This divine connection brings about peace, clarity, and alignment with His purposes.

Additionally, Jesus Himself declared in John 12:32 (NIV), "And I, when I am lifted up from the earth, will draw all people to Myself." This profound statement illuminates the captivating nature of worship and praise centered on Jesus. When we exalt Him with authenticity and wholeheartedness, we create an environment where His presence permeates our lives, beckoning others to encounter His transformative love.

Engaging in the discipline of worship and praise allows us to embrace our true purpose and satisfy the deep longing within us to commune with our Creator. In this sacred space, we find restoration, peace, and a profound sense of belonging. As we lift up Jesus, our minds are renewed, our spirits are invigorated, and we are filled to overflowing with His abundant presence.

Let us wholeheartedly embrace the disciplines of prayer, reading the word, waiting on the Lord, and worshiping him. Open your *Heart Journey*™ *Journal* and work on your **Individual Heartwork - Cede to Spiritual Discipline.**

## CEDE TO OBEDIENCE

In the journey of restoring lost opportunities, one crucial step stands out: the discipline of obedience to the Lord. While it may be technically categorized as a spiritual discipline, I want to emphasize its profound significance.

Let us turn to our friend Deborah again, who grew up in a family where most of her relatives abused alcohol, which led to violence and trauma. As a coping strategy, Deborah drank compulsively and used drugs as a teen until she met Jesus. As she came into relationship with Him, He spoke to her, "If you want what I have for you, you will lay this down." In her love for Him, she did lay down alcohol and drugs. Much later in life, a friend of Deborah's encouraged her to try wine, and encouraged her to moderate through her long-standing relationship with Jesus. This seemed reasonable to Deborah, and she started drinking wine socially. However, it was not long before her relationship with wine became compulsive, and her peace was elusive. After several months of struggle, she sought the Lord for victory, and He said, "Go back to what I told you long ago." She again laid down alcohol, and her peace returned. Deborah's story highlights that obedience is directly tied to our peace and our purpose. We cannot walk in restoration and disobedience at the same time.

Now, let me ask you a pivotal question: Do you truly desire to embrace God's best for your life? The psalmist beautifully declares in Psalm 34:8 (NRSCV), "O taste and see that the Lord is good; happy are those who take refuge in Him." This truth deeply resonates within my heart. I yearn for every good thing He has in store for me and to live out His divine plans in this earthly existence. Do you share this same longing? If so, I implore you to consider what God is calling you to release. Is there something He is gently urging you to lay down, whispering, "If you want to experience what I have for you, let go of this burden"? Beloved, I assure you that it is safe to surrender it. In fact, holding onto it is far riskier than releasing it. Your healing will spring forth with remarkable swiftness, just as Isaiah 58 assures us.

I invite you to open your *Heart Journey™ Journal* and reflect on where God is summoning you to walk in more refined obedience. Complete your **Individual Heartwork - Cede to Obedience.**

## CEDE TO GOD'S LOVE

One more vital aspect that calls for our ceding is surrendering to God's boundless love, and a beautiful pathway to do so is by immersing ourselves in His affection for us. The truth of 1 John 4:19 (KJV) resonates deeply within our hearts: "We love Him because He first loved us." It is our aim to not only receive that overwhelming love, but also to extend it to others in our lives. However, it is important to recognize that often, we try to give away a love we have not fully embraced ourselves. Thus, we must take intentional steps to deepen our understanding and experience of God's love.

Set aside moments of reflection to think about and ponder on the depth of God's love. Engage in reading and meditating upon the Scriptures that speak of His love, allowing His word to permeate your heart and mind. Visualize His love with your holy imagination, allowing the imagery to bring a tangible sense of His affection and care. Let the knowledge of His love seep into every corner of your being, filling you to the point of intoxication, as described in Ephesians 5:18.

Now take some time in your *Heart Journey™ Journal* and complete **Individual Heartwork - Cede to God's Love.**

## CEDE TO LISTENING TO YOUR WHOLE SELF

In our journey of growth and restoration, another essential aspect we must cede to is the practice of listening to our whole selves—our body, soul, and spirit. While we have already discussed the significance of listening to the Holy Spirit and obeying His guidance, let us now explore additional ways to attune to our true selves. Remember that our true self is the self as God intended, not the sinful nature.

Throughout this journey, you have invested considerable effort in nurturing your relationship with yourself, and it is crucial to continue this practice. By regularly and prayerfully checking in with your emotions and body throughout the day, you create moments of fellowship with Jesus, inviting His presence and guidance into your inner world. This practice cultivates a deeper connection with Him and opens the door to His healing and transformative work in your life. Consider setting a timer on your phone as a gentle reminder to engage in self-check-ins. By embracing this practice more intentionally, you will experience fewer instances of unresolved trauma or distress lingering and building up in your daily life. It is important to prayerfully acknowledge and be present with what is going on within us, rather than ignoring or suppressing it.

When we consciously engage with our body sensations, approaching them with loving intention and the knowledge that Jesus is with us in our bodies, we find liberation. Embrace an attentive connection with your body, resisting the temptation to dissociate or detach from it. Allow yourself to fully embody all the parts of your true self with Jesus.

Additionally, I want to encourage you to incorporate the use of your RESOURCE™ skills on a daily basis. These skills are not limited to trauma work alone; they are meant to be used as daily life tools. Take proactive steps to keep your mind healthy, practice self-nurturing, utilize tracking and grounding techniques, and engage in Christian relaxation exercises. Integrate these skills into your daily routine as preventative measures and use them as needed. Keep them at the forefront of your awareness. And remember to prioritize self-care, ensuring that it becomes an integral part of your self-care plan.

In addition, reflect on what self-care truly means to you. Are there areas in your life where you need to play more? Many of us may have missed out on sufficient opportunities for play during our formative years, and it is vital to make room for joyful recreation. Incorporating regular playtime into your self-care plan is essential. Fun, even in small doses, is powerful and needed in our daily lives.[32]

Another significant aspect of listening to our whole selves is acknowledging and embracing grief. Throughout our journey, we have focused on completing and integrating past traumas and losses, often encountering moments where frozen emotions resurface, leading to a sense of grief. It is important to recognize that feeling grief is actually a positive sign, as it brings us closer to wholeness and health. As noted earlier in our study, grief is like a candle that we cannot bypass; we must allow it to burn down. When there is loss, grief and mourning are the natural expressions of our hearts. If you are experiencing grief, strive to manage it in a healthy manner by making time for processing. Seek ways to empower and comfort yourself during this process. It is essential to surrender to the season of grieving when necessary, recognizing it is for your ultimate benefit.

Deborah shares her own experiences of feeling weary in the midst of grieving a familial suicide. Yet, as the weight of grief lifted, she discovered true joy and a greater capacity to embrace positive emotions. Allowing ourselves to fully experience the challenging feelings not only facilitates growth and healing, but also expands our ability to experience joy and happiness.

Reflecting on my personal journey, I recall a time when I focused on strengthening my weak and aching hips through weightlifting. Despite experiencing discomfort during the weightlifting, I realized my hips would continue to hurt whether I worked on strengthening them or not. The pain I endured while working out was instrumental in building strength and ultimately decreasing pain. Similarly, grief follows a similar pattern. The pain endured during the grieving process strengthens and transforms us. It is pain on the way up and out. If you find that you are getting stuck in grief, it is crucial to seek professional help and support. We do not want to remain trapped in a perpetual state of grief, but we also should not fear or avoid it entirely.

Now, take some dedicated time to journal and reflect on all the elements we have discussed in your **Individual Heartwork - Cede to Listening to Your Whole Self.**

## CEDE TO A NEW NARRATIVE

In this segment, we embark on a transformative journey of Ceding to a New Narrative, intricately intertwined with our Reframe skill and narrative work. As we alter the story we tell ourselves, we breathe new life into our existence. Consider how you perceive yourself, communicate about yourself, and think about yourself. Throughout this profound healing transformation, you have undergone a remarkable metamorphosis. It is now time for your self-perception and self-expression to align with this growth.

Remember, our words and thoughts carry immense power, echoing ceaselessly into the world like ripples in a vast ocean of possibilities. In the Bible, our thoughts and words are highlighted as powerful forces that shape our realities. Proverbs 18:21 (AMP) states, "Death and life are in the power of the tongue," emphasizing the significant impact our words have on our lives. Similarly, we have noted that Romans 12:2 urges believers to renew their minds and be transformed, recognizing the power of our thoughts in influencing our actions and experiences.

Now that we have renovated your heart home, what narrative are you weaving about yourself? What narrative are you painting for your life? It is time for a transformative shift. Are you speaking in alignment with God's truth about who you are? Are you affirming, "I am a cherished princess, a beloved daughter of the King"? Are you allowing yourself to truly feel the depth of these words, speaking them and internalizing them until they become an intrinsic part of your being?

Your words have the potential to shape your reality. Embrace the authority of biblical affirmations and the profound impact they can have on your self-perception, your thoughts, and your emotions. Embrace the fullness of your identity as a beloved child of God. Let your renewed narrative be a catalyst for empowerment, joy, and a deep sense of purpose.

Complete your *Heart Journey*™ *Journal,* assignment **Individual Heartwork - Cede to a New Narrative.**

## CEDE TO JOY

After going through the process of healing and getting rid of deep-rooted trauma, it is time to fully embrace the idea of giving in to joy. In Nehemiah 8:10 (NRSV), we are reminded not to let sadness overwhelm us because the joy we find in the Lord is what gives us strength. "The joy of the Lord is your strength." This powerful verse reminds us that, no matter what trials and difficulties we face, we have the ability to experience genuine joy in the presence of the Lord, and it is through His unwavering strength that we are carried. As the African American spiritual verbalizes so well, "You can have all of this world, just give me Jesus."

Walking in joy is not some abstract or elusive concept that only happens on special occasions. As believers, we have the amazing ability to cultivate and embrace the Lord's joy within us as a daily way of life. It is not dependent on our external circumstances, but is rooted in our unshakeable relationship with God. Reflect on the example of Jesus: despite being aware of the immense suffering that awaited Him, He did not succumb to dread. Consider the incredible nature of this truth. Jesus possessed knowledge of the hardships He would face, yet He remained full of joy. And just as Jesus experienced joy amidst adversity, we, too, can embrace and radiate joy, Beloved. The joy we possess is not temporary or fleeting but firmly anchored in the eternal promises and overflowing love of our Heavenly Father, whose Spirit is literally within us. There is no limit to how filled with Him we can live today and every day, if we hunger, surrender, and believe. His kingdom is within you (Luke 17:20-21).

When we make the choice to embrace joy, we are making a conscious decision to shift our focus from life's burdens to the goodness and faithfulness of God. We learn to celebrate His presence in every aspect of our journey, finding joy in His provision, His guidance, and His unchanging love for us. It is a joyful surrender, an acknowledgment of the indescribable joy that comes from knowing we are deeply cherished and cared for by the Creator of the universe, and because of that, all is well.

Giving in to joy does not mean we ignore or downplay the hardships we face. Instead, it empowers us to rise above our circumstances, allowing the joy of the Lord to become our source of potency and might. It is an active pursuit of finding beauty in the midst of trials which we are promised we will face. But we can discover gratitude in every season and choose to bask in the radiance of God's joyful presence.

Open your *Heart Journey*™ *Journal* and complete your **Individual Heartwork - Cede to Joy and then enjoy the Radiant Memories Activity** in your journal.

Use this QR code to access audible versions of activities.

## TASTE GOODNESS DAILY

Tasting the goodness of the Lord daily is an integral part of embracing joy, which aligns with our current focus on the "T" in our RECONSTRUCTION acronym, "Taste Goodness Daily." When we have experienced hurt and trauma, our natural instinct is to dwell on the negative and build defenses to protect ourselves. However, we must learn to strike a balance and not solely gravitate toward negative and depressive thoughts. It is time to choose to live a life of restored joy and opportunities. We are changing our narratives from those who are victims, to those who have all we need for life and godliness (2 Peter 1:3).

Just as there is a trauma whirlpool that can pull us toward negativity, there is also a counter wind within us that draws us toward positivity and healing (John 3:8). Our goal is to expand our capacity for joy, peace, excitement, love, and contentment through our connection with Jesus. To achieve this, we need to strengthen our neural pathways toward the positive, and spiritually nourish them through practice and conscious effort. We submit to thinking the thoughts of Christ, as neurons that fire together wire together.[33] Hence, the more we focus on positive thoughts and savor uplifting experiences, the more we reinforce those pathways. We do not want the negative aspects to dominate our neural pathways; instead, we aim for a faith-filled focus on the positive while remaining authentic.

Barbara Frederickson's current research on happiness reveals that we need a ratio of three positive emotions to every negative emotion in order to thrive.[34] This applies not only to our interactions with others, but also to our self-talk.

We do not ignore or suppress negative emotions, but we strive to increase the positive, according to Philippians 4:8 (ESV). "Finally, brothers, whatever is true, whatever is honorable, whatever is just, whatever is pure, whatever is lovely, whatever is commendable, if there is any excellence, if there is anything worthy of praise, think about these things." It is important to let go of learned helplessness, a belief that we have no control over our lives or the ability to improve our circumstances. Remember, although we cannot change others, we must own that we can change ourselves.

In essence, we aim to be pragmatic optimists, understanding the benefits of being realistic yet full of faith. Optimists tend to enjoy better physical and mental health outcomes and longer lives overall. By maintaining hope in God's goodness in our present lives, we open ourselves up to participate in the restoration of lost opportunities. This involves identifying what traumas or unmet needs have taken away from us and working alongside Jesus to reclaim those opportunities.

## RECLAIMING LOST OPPORTUNITIES

Throughout this study, we have diligently focused on the transformative power of Jesus, who graciously gives us back what was stolen from us. Our holy imagination has been a vital tool in this process, allowing us to envision the restoration and redemption Jesus longs to bring into our lives. Now, we are taking concrete steps and actively participating with Jesus in beautifying our lives and reclaiming what was lost.

Our journey has not been easy, and we have walked through deep waters. But now it is time to enjoy the fruit of your labors. 1 Peter 5:10 (ESV) states, "And after you have suffered a little while, the God of all grace, who has called you to His eternal glory in Christ, will Himself restore, confirm, strengthen, and establish you." This verse assures us that God, in His grace, not only restores what was taken from us, but also strengthens and establishes us in the process. Our active participation in reclaiming lost opportunities aligns with God's desire to bring restoration and establish us in His abundant blessings.

## DEBORAH'S STORY

For instance, Deborah shared her desire to have participated in competitive sports, but was hindered by fear and anxiety stemming from her home life. However, through her *Heart Journey*™ work, Deborah experienced profound healing. She discovered the excitement of reclaiming lost opportunities and realized she could still take tennis lessons. Although hesitant at first, she confronted and overcame her fears, recognizing that nothing could now hold her back except herself. Deborah started playing tennis and relished the Lord's restoration of those lost opportunities.

Now, it is your turn to reflect on your narratives from Chapter Five and identify the lost opportunities in your life. Begin working with Jesus through your **Individual Heartwork - Reclaiming Lost Opportunities**, allowing Him to guide you in reclaiming what has been taken away. You will have three exercises to complete, including one that will reclaim lost opportunities, one that transforms your fear into faith, and another that increases the joy in your life. Embrace the transformative journey of tasting God's goodness as you participate in the restoration of those precious moments and experiences.

Also, take time to complete the **Individual Heartwork questions and Heart Group Discussion** work included in your journal.

Beloved, I am beaming with pride over your amazing tenacity in this study! Every bit of work will pay off. And you really can enjoy your life, even with the ups and downs. You can do this, Beloved!

I look forward to seeing you in the next chapter, where we will discover and launch into your life purpose in a way that honors your traumas that are healing.

## LET US PRAY.

Heavenly Father,

You have done such an amazing work in our heart home during this journey. We have learned so much about ourselves—every part of our beings, how life experiences affected us, and how we can become and remain overcomers. Thank You, Father, for walking with us on this journey. May our hearts and minds continue to be open to Your heart's desire for every aspect of our lives, and may we continue to embrace Your healing touch.

In Jesus' name, Amen.

# *Chapter*

## ELEVEN

### Restoring My Purpose

*Instead of your shame you will receive a double portion, and instead of disgrace you will rejoice in your inheritance.*

*And so you will inherit a double portion in your land, and everlasting joy will be yours.*

**Isaiah 61:7 (NIV)**

You have always had God's thread of unique destiny woven through your life. Now it is time to discover or rediscover that destiny and to learn how to operate more fully, more joyfully from that place of flow and efficacy! This chapter will get you there. We will also discover renewed skills for relating to others, while living from a whole self and enjoying a full bouquet of life! Moreover, you will personally encounter streams of living water flowing from the very scars that once marked your wounds!

We have journeyed together so far on this transformative *Heart Journey*™, and now we stand at a significant juncture where we can assess and embrace the glorious purpose that God has for our lives. Our ultimate aim is to live in alignment with His perfect will. Along this journey, we have gathered a diverse set of tools that will empower you to navigate future trials and challenges with resilience. Whether faced with loss, triggered traumas, or other obstacles, you now possess the means to address these situations effectively. From satisfying unmet needs to reversing the impact of past trauma, healing boundary ruptures, and releasing the burdens of resentment, you have a range of strategies at your disposal to triumph over these hurdles.

As we approach the culmination of this profound healing journey, the vision of our destiny and purpose becomes clearer than ever. Our heart home has been meticulously reconstructed using the finest materials, infused with the presence of the Lord at every turn. Yet, our work is not complete. Now, it is time to fill our heart home not only with joy, cheerfulness, and discipline but also with a purpose that flows from the depths of our being. There is a unique, God-assigned purpose that wants to emanate from within each of us, transforming us and impacting the world around us. In our RECONSTRUCTION™ acronym, we now come to "I" for "Inventory Purpose."

Throughout this study, we have explored Deborah's story. We have also spent ample time in John 7:38 (NIV), which says "Whoever believes in Me, as Scripture has said, rivers of living water will flow from within them." The word "river" can mean torrent. Today, Deborah, whose heart has been transformed through going through the *Heart Journey*™ study, ministers to others in the very areas in which she was once devastated. Jesus has transformed her trauma wounds into torrents of living water that flow from Deborah in the very places the enemy tried to devastate her. He has done this in Deborah's life, in my life, in billions of women's lives, and He will do this for you as well!

The Father longs to take your deepest traumas and transform them into powerful streams of living water. Your sufferings have the potential to be woven into the fabric of your destiny. Nothing is ever truly lost; nothing is beyond the Master's magnificent ability to redeem and repurpose. Every ounce of pain and heartache can be beautifully interwoven into the tapestry of your purpose, becoming a legacy gift that impacts the world around you. The enemy may have plotted against you, but God's counter assignment prevails, turning every scheme into raw material for the masterpiece He is crafting through your life.

We have indeed cleared away vast amounts of wreckage the enemy had brought against you. The very areas where he has attacked you, the places that have caused deep wounds within your soul, are often the same places where you will minister most powerfully. It is within those very depths of pain and vulnerability that a river of living water can spring forth, bringing forth remarkable life and touching the lives of many around you.

Let us delve into the remarkable story of Corrie ten Boom, as a powerful example. Her life indeed carried a profound message of the transformative power of forgiveness, which originated from the very place where she had experienced deep wounding. Corrie ten Boom endured unimaginable suffering and loss during the Holocaust, enduring the horrors of a concentration camp alongside her sister, whom she loved more than life itself.

One pivotal moment in Corrie ten Boom's life occurred during a church service where she was preaching. A man approached her, a former Nazi officer who had played a significant role in her sister's death while they were both in the concentration camp. This man extended his hand, seeking reconciliation. In that moment, Corrie turned to the Lord, acknowledging her own inadequacy to forgive this man. It was an agonizing moment when time stood still, as she battled with immense hatred for this man who took her sister, her main comfort in the camps, and caused so much inhumane brutality. After what seemed like hours, she beseeched the Lord for His forgiveness to flow through her, knowing she could not forgive in her own strength. As she reached out her hand in obedience, she was suddenly flooded with a palpable presence of the warm and engulfing love and forgiveness of the Lord. By His strength and grace, she embraced reconciliation with the very person who had caused her immense trauma and pain.

This profound act of obedience and healing became the defining message of Corrie ten Boom's life. From the depths of her wounded heart, she emerged as a powerful minister of grace and healing, impacting countless lives with her message of love and reconciliation.

Corrie ten Boom's life serves as a testament to the torrents of living water that can arise from the depths of our own pain, through Jesus. Similarly, your own experiences of pain and struggle have equipped you with a unique empathy and understanding. The very wounds that have caused you to cry out to God become the source from which compassion and life-giving words flow. As you embrace the healing and restoration brought by God's love, the scars of your past become a testimony of His redeeming power. He will flow through you in these very places of pain. Just as Jesus' scars have become power and love to the world, through Him, so will yours.

Remember, it is in our weakness that God's strength is made perfect (2 Corinthians 12:9). The places where we have encountered our deepest hurts become the fertile ground for seeds of hope to take root. Just as a wounded heart, once healed, becomes a beacon of light for others who are walking in darkness, your story and journey hold the potential to inspire and uplift those who may be facing similar trials. Psalm 40 mentions how God hears our cries and plants our feet on solid ground.

*I waited patiently for the Lord; He turned to me and heard my cry. He lifted me out of the slimy pit, out of the mud and mire; He set my feet on a rock and gave me a firm place to stand.*

*He put a new song in my mouth, a hymn of praise to our God. Many will see and fear the Lord and put their trust in Him.*

### Psalms 40:1-3 (NIV)

## VISION BOARD: CHRISTIAN VERSION

In this chapter, we will investigate your purpose through various means. Proverbs 25:2 (NIV) says, "It is the glory of God to conceal a matter; to search out a matter is the glory of kings." We will search out the matter of your purpose! To start, we will have you delve into the creative part of your soul as well as the mind of the Spirit to create a vision board.

A vision board is a powerful tool that allows us to visualize our God-inspired dreams and aspirations. It serves as a tangible representation of the desires and goals we hold in our hearts. As we embark on the journey of creating a vision board by the guidance of the Holy Spirit, we approach this process with a spirit of prayerfulness and surrender, trusting that the Lord will direct our steps.

It is important to recognize that God's plans for us will surpass our own limited expectations. He invites us to dream big with Him and to embrace the lavish vision He has for our lives. Therefore, as you engage in this activity, maintain an attitude of openness and faith before the Lord. Here, we choose to lean not on our own understanding but to place our trust in the Lord's big vision for our lives. We acknowledge that His wisdom surpasses ours and that He holds the key to unlocking the fullness of our potential. As Proverbs 3:5-6 reminds us, we commit to trusting Him in all our ways, knowing that He will make our paths straight. He will always call us to places that will require faith and His power. So, the call will always surpass our abilities.

Beloved, all we have worked toward is culminating into launching you into a life filled with His purpose for you. Open Your *Heart Journey*™ *Journal* to Chapter Eleven and complete your **Individual Heartwork - Vision Board: Christian Version**. I am thrilled that we are embarking on a journey to discover and live out God's purpose for our lives.

## GOD'S PURPOSE WOVEN THROUGH TIME

Did you know there is a book written about you that reveals God's perfect purpose for every single day of your life? Psalm 139:16 affirms that all your days were written by Him in His book. Wow! It is incredible to think that God has a purpose book specifically tailored to you for each day of your life, and your responsibility is to align yourself with His intentions each day. His purpose has always been interwoven within the very fabric of your being. By studying your life, your interests, passions, and the stirrings of your heart over time, we can uncover more of the purpose that God has always laid out for you.

It is important to note that God's purpose for you is not limited by the seasons of your life, including any time before you became a Christian. Each person is uniquely stamped with purpose by God, and He activates that purpose through His Spirit when one receives Him. Your journey, even before your faith, has significance and can provide valuable insights into the destiny God has planned for you.

For example, our friend Deborah received Jesus as her Lord and Savior at the age of nineteen, yet even before that time she had a desire to teach and encourage others throughout her life. She even used to line up her stuffed animals and teach and encourage them as a young child. In the midst of her living her life for herself, God's unique purpose, written into her, was tattooed upon her heart. Romans 11:29 (ESV) says, "For the gifts and the calling of God are irrevocable." This will be true for you as well.

So, as we continue on this journey of discovering your purpose, let us remain open to the leading of the Holy Spirit. We will now inventory your interests, passions, temperament, gifts, talents, and the like over time at each age and stage of your life. Through this exercise we will decode more of the brilliant purpose that God planned for you since before your conception (Jeremiah 1:5)!

Open your *Heart Journey Journal* to Chapter Eleven, and complete your **Individual Heartwork - God's Purpose Woven through Time.**

Beloved, you are a masterpiece intricately crafted by God's loving hands. You are not only a masterpiece in and of yourself, but you are also a vital piece of the larger puzzle that is God's universal and masterful plan to seek and to save all that is lost. He designed you with intention and distinctive purpose, and your unique calling and mission intersect and connect profoundly with the lives of others.

Within the depths of your beautiful being, God has selectively and tenderly placed spiritual gifts and sought-out talents that are designed to be shared with others as unparalleled gems to the world. Let us explore your spiritual gifts as part of decoding your delightful purpose inheritance from your Father.

## SPIRITUAL GIFTS

The Word of God, specifically in 1 Corinthians 12, 13, and 14, speaks extensively about the various spiritual gifts bestowed upon believers. It is through this exploration that we can gain insights into the unique abilities and callings that God has placed within us. Below is an in-exhaustive list of spiritual gifts in Scripture.

Each of these spiritual gifts serves a distinctive purpose within the body of Christ. They are given by the Holy Spirit to equip believers for service, to edify and strengthen the church, and to advance the Kingdom of God. As we discover and operate in our spiritual gifts, we fulfill our calling and contribute to the harmonious functioning of the body, working together for the glory of God and the benefit of others.

1. Administration - 1 Corinthians 12:28 (NIV): "those with gifts of administration."

2.  Apostleship* - Ephesians 4:11(NIV): "So Christ Himself gave the apostles."

3.  Creative communication - Exodus 31:3-5(NIV): "I have filled him with the Spirit of God, with wisdom, with understanding, with knowledge and with all kinds of skills."

4.  Deliverance - Mark 16:17 (NIV): "And these signs will accompany those who believe: In My name, they will drive out demons."

5.  Discipleship - Matthew 28:19-20 (NIV): "Therefore go and make disciples of all nations."

6.  Distinguishing between spirits – 1 Corinthians 12:8 (NIV): "to another distinguishing between spirits"

7.  Encouragement - Romans 12:8 (NIV): "if it is to encourage, then give encouragement."

8.  Evangelism - Ephesians 4:11 (NIV): "So Christ Himself gave the apostles, the prophets, the evangelists."

9.  Faith - 1 Corinthians 12:9 (NIV): "to another faith."

10. Giving - Romans 12:8 (NIV): "if it is to give, do it generously."

11. Healing - 1 Corinthians 12:9 (NIV): "gifts of healing."

12. Help - 1 Corinthians 12:28 (NIV): "those able to help others."

13. Hospitality - Romans 12:13 (NIV): "Practice hospitality."

14. Intercession - Romans 8:26 (NIV): "The Spirit helps us in our weakness. We do not know what we ought to pray for, but the Spirit Himself* intercedes for us through wordless groans."

15. Interpretation of tongues* - 1 Corinthians 12:10 (NIV): "to another the interpretation of tongues."

16. Knowledge - 1 Corinthians 12:8 (NIV): "to another a message of knowledge."

17. Leadership - Romans 12:8 (NIV): "if it is to lead, do it diligently."

18. Mercy - Romans 12:8 (NIV): "if it is to show mercy, do it cheerfully."

19. Miracles* - 1 Corinthians 12:10 (NIV): "to another miraculous powers."

20. Music/worship - 1 Chronicles 25:1-3 (NIV): "to prophesy accompanied by the lyres, harps, and cymbals."

21. Pastoring/Shepherding - Ephesians 4:11 (NIV): "So Christ Himself gave the apostles, the prophets, the evangelists, the pastors and teachers."

22. Prophecy* - 1 Corinthians 12:10 (NIV): "to another prophecy."

23. Serving - 1 Peter 4:10-11 (NIV): "Each of you should use whatever gift you have received to serve others."

24. Teaching - Romans 12:7 (NIV): "if it is teaching, then teach."

25. Tongues* - 1 Corinthians 12:10 (NIV): "to another speaking in different kinds of tongues."

26. Wisdom - 1 Corinthians 12:8 (NIV): "to another the message of wisdom."

*Note: Some denominations believe that certain gifts, marked with an asterisk, have passed away or are not actively present in the Church today. These beliefs vary among different theological perspectives.

You will be exploring your gifts in your Heartwork. Discovering and utilizing your spiritual gifts allows you to walk in alignment with your God-given purpose and more poignantly impact the lives of others.

Deborah, through her *Heart Journey*™ process, discovered gifts of teaching, mercy, and prophecy that seem to flow from her when she ministers in her small group. Similarly, I have discovered that my main gifts include encouragement, teaching, and healing of the heart. These gifts flow through me as I serve others in the church. It is essential to identify your own spiritual gifts and recognize how they align with your purpose and the needs of those around you.

Now open your *Heart Journey*™ *Journal* to Chapter Eleven and complete your **Individual Heartwork - My Spiritual Gifts.**

## MY PURPOSE STATEMENT

All your work thus far has positioned you to launch into your purpose. Creating a purpose statement is an invaluable practice for us as we seek to align our lives with God's marvelous, personalized, and uniquely designed plan for each of us. Beloved, you are a supernova event, a once-in-a-lifetime marvel that will never, ever happen again. No one will ever possess your gifts, talents, experiences, personality, flow, appearance, temperament, equipping, and flare all wrapped into one God-sized package ever again. Consider, dear one, the vital importance of stepping into your purpose. You are a one-of-a-kind gift to the world, fashioned by your Creator for such a time as this! The world needs you, and the body of Christ is yearning for you to step into the fullness of your calling.

"When I run, I feel God's pleasure"—these powerful words spoken by Eric Liddell in the movie *Chariots of Fire* resonate deeply with those of us who have discovered the wonder of living a life on purpose. It is a profound declaration that encapsulates the incredible joy and fulfillment that comes from aligning our lives with God's plan for us.

To feel God's pleasure is to experience a deep sense of oneness, connection, and affirmation from our Heavenly Father. It is a tangible manifestation of His delight in seeing us fulfill the purpose He has uniquely designed for us. Just as Eric Liddell felt God's pleasure when he ran, each one of us can experience that divine affirmation when we wholeheartedly pursue our God-given passions and talents.

So, when do we feel God's pleasure? It is in those moments when we are fully engaged in activities that align with our purpose. It could be in the midst of using our gifts to serve others, when we lose track of time because we are so engrossed in doing what we love. It may be when we are passionately pursuing a cause or endeavor that resonates with the very core of our being. It could be in acts of kindness and compassion in which we can tangibly embody the heart of Christ, feeling His love flowing through us and touching the lives of others. It could even be in quiet moments of prayer and worship when we feel His presence surrounding us.

Feeling God's pleasure is not limited to grand accomplishments or extraordinary feats. It can also be found in the ordinary moments of our lives, when we bring our whole, spirit-filled selves to whatever we do, seeking to honor and glorify God in all things. For example, consider the mother who has a child with special needs and who requires homebound care much of the time. Oh, how Jesus honors the gift and sacrifice this mother is giving to her child in the secret place of a life laid down.

Living a life on purpose is a marvelous gift from God. It fills our hearts with a deep sense of meaning, fulfillment, and joy. When we embrace our purpose, we discover that we are part of a grand tapestry of living stones woven by the Creator Himself (1 Peter 2:4-5). In science, we know that the sum is greater than its parts; similarly as we step into our purpose, we help equip everyone around us to flow in purpose, as we move together by the Spirit of God.

The Scripture announces, "For we are His workmanship, created in Christ Jesus for good works, which God prepared beforehand, that we should walk in them" (Ephesians 2:10, ESV). In addition, the Scripture says, "For just as each of us has one body with many members, and these members do not all have the same function, so in Christ we, though many, form one body, and each member belongs to all the others" (Romans 12:4-5, NIV). We are made to step into purpose while remaining interconnected within the body of Christ.

Dear friend, when you align yourself with His unique plan for you, you will not only feel His pleasure, but you will also witness the transformative power of a life lived on purpose. Now open your *Heart Journey™ Journal* to Chapter Eleven and complete your **Individual Heartwork - God's Purpose Woven Through Time, - My Spiritual Gifts,** and **- My Purpose Statement.**

## OPERATE FROM PURPOSE

Now we come to "O" in our RECONSTRUCTION acronym, which stands for "Operate from Purpose." In order to operate from purpose, you need to know what your purpose is and activate your faith by shaking off fear and failure. In this segment, you will shake off the dust of fear and failure, and in your *Heart Journey™ Journal,* you will go through an exercise that will activate your faith.

## SHAKE OFF THE DUST

Beloved, imagine what you could accomplish with Jesus and the right team if you were not afraid of failure. Let us recall the Scriptures from Matthew 10 where Jesus encourages the disciples to shake the dust off their feet if they are not welcomed in a home or town. That word "shake" means to violently shake.

*"Whatever town or village you enter, search there
for some worthy person and stay at their house until you leave.
As you enter the home, give it your greeting. If the home is deserving,
let your peace rest on it; if it is not, let your peace return to you.
If anyone will not welcome you or listen to your words, leave that home
or town and shake the dust off your feet."*

**Matthew 10:11-14 (NIV)**

Dear one, ask yourself, "What do I need to violently shake off in regard to fulfilling my purpose? Is there a mindset, a fear of failure, or an attitude of helplessness that I have held onto for a long time, like a security blanket?" It is now time to let it go. The boulders have been moved away through Christ, and you can move forward, unobstructed by fear, into purpose.

Open your *Heart Journey*™ *Journal* to Chapter Eleven and complete your **Individual Heartwork - Shake off the Dust and enjoy this activity: Visualize His Purpose Fulfilled**

Use this QR code to access audible versions of activities.

## HEALING THROUGH ACTION

In the midst of the tragic loss of His cousin, John the Baptist, Jesus, seeking solace, invited His disciples to a quiet place to find rest. However, even in His grief, Jesus found Himself surrounded by a multitude of people. Despite His broken heart, Jesus performed a miracle by multiplying bread and fish to feed the crowd. This scene teaches us that healing does not always come from withdrawing and seeking comfort with loved ones; sometimes healing comes when we step out and engage in the work of God.

Isaiah 58 speaks of the healing that comes as we reach out and give to others. True healing and purpose can be discovered as we humbly follow God's lead, even amidst our own pain, and engage in selfless actions. In Proverbs 3:5-6, we are reminded to trust in the Lord with all our hearts and lean not on our own understanding. By surrendering to Him and allowing Him to lead us, we can walk in alignment with His purpose for our lives despite our circumstances.

While we may feel our own journey is not yet complete, the truth is that we will not experience the reality of full sanctification in this earthly life. Therefore, part of our healing lies in moving forward and embracing our destiny. God's call is always forward moving, so it is important to gain clarity on his purpose for our lives and make any necessary changes now. We can find comfort and encouragement in Jeremiah 29:11, knowing that God has plans for our future, plans to prosper us and not to harm us.

To strengthen your commitment to on-purpose living, consider finding an accountability partner who can provide support and hold you accountable to walking in destiny. Share your vision and calling with trusted friends who can walk alongside you and offer their wisdom and encouragement through obstacles.

As we navigate setbacks and failures along the way, we can draw inspiration from the concept of "failing forward" coined by John

Maxwell. It means that we learn from our failures, rise above them, and keep moving forward with determination and persistence. Failure is a normal part of forward movement.

Give yourself grace and space to make mistakes along the way. Embrace the truth that being flawed is part of being fabulous, for it is through our weaknesses that God's power shines brightest (2 Corinthians 12:9). In Matthew 11:28-30, Jesus invites us to take His yoke upon us and learn from Him, for His yoke is easy and His burden is light. By following Him wholeheartedly and embracing the unforced rhythms of grace, we can find rest and fulfillment in living on purpose by His Spirit.

Open your *Heart Journey*™ *Journal* to Chapter Eleven and complete your **Individual Heartwork - Operating from Purpose.**

## NAVIGATING RELATIONSHIPS ANEW

As we explore the final letter of our RECONSTRUCTION acronym, "N" for "Navigate Relationships Anew," we celebrate in the healing we have experienced on this journey. Yet, with all our accomplishments, there are likely still patterns in our relationships that are not healthy, often driven by ingrained habits. This segment will give us a few tools to renew our minds in our relationships.

God has fashioned us for healthy relationships. He desires for us to break free from old patterns and embrace new, healing designs in our relationships. Oh, the freedom He wants to bring! Recall again that in Romans 12:2 (NIV), we are reminded: "Do not conform to the pattern of this world, but be transformed by the renewing of your mind." By cultivating self-awareness of our patterns and surrendering to the transformative work of the Lord in those areas, we can liberate ourselves from destructive cycles and embark on a journey of healthier communication and relationships.

Object relations theories teach us that our childhood experiences create patterns that can be unconsciously relived in our adult relationships. These patterns, such as the dynamics between an angry parent and a scapegoated child, can profoundly impact our ability to cultivate healthy connections. Recognizing and addressing our trauma patterns are essential. Just as an adult woman would not attempt to wear clothes from her elementary school days, we want to recognize and step out of old patterns and "put on" new ways of relating.

## DEBORAH'S STORY

We can again learn from Deborah's experience. She recognized that her past patterns with her father had influenced her relationships. She was terrified of how he pursued her with rage and neediness as a child. In reaction to this, she tended to be drawn to those who were highly avoidant in attachment style and who would betray her rather than pursue her. However, she used her *Heart Journey*™ tools to boldly face patterns with her father and began to relate more rightly to others, especially in the romantic arena.

As we navigate relationships, it is crucial to stay off the Triangle of Pain, avoiding victimhood, scapegoating, anger, or over-caretaking. Instead, let us relate to others as adults, each carrying our own load and supporting one another when needed. Let us be thoughtful, living out our values rather than reacting impulsively. As you continue on this segment, you will have the opportunity to explore and align your actions with your values, allowing them to guide your relationships.

We want to live out of our values and not out of our pain. We want to live from God's Spirit and not on the Tringle of Pain. In your *Heart Journey*™ *Journal* Heartwork for this segment, you identify the values you want to live from in your relationships.

## CORE NEGATIVE IMAGE

In our relationships, we sometimes carry deep-seated perceptions and beliefs about ourselves and others that originate from past wounds. Dr. Terry Real, a renowned family therapist, refers to "core negative images."[35] These images can significantly impact how we view and engage with our loved ones, often leading to misunderstandings and gridlocked conflict. This concept is similar to object relations theory.

Core negative images have a way of distorting our interpretations of others' intentions and actions. They cause us to project past hurts and fears into current situations with others, as we are triggered by our own emotional responses that are disproportionate to reality. When we acknowledge the impact of past wounds on our present interactions, we gain the ability to separate our current experiences from the lingering effects of unresolved childhood pain. This self-awareness empowers us to respond to our loved ones with empathy and understanding, breaking free from the repetitive patterns of the past.

## DEBORAH'S STORY

In her *Heart Journey*™, Deborah learned that when her husband tried to express a concern about their relationship, Deborah found herself becoming defensive, interpreting his words as blame. It became clear that her reaction was influenced by a core negative image she held of him as an angry parent. Through her Heartwork, Deborah realized that around 75 percent of her reaction was rooted in her own image of her father from childhood, while only about 25 percent related to the actual situation. This realization served as a powerful reminder of the significance of healing and transforming these negative images.

Navigating these core negative images calls for patience, self-reflection, and open communication. It requires us to explore our personal triggers and wounds while extending understanding to those we hold dear. As we embark on this journey of healing and growth, let us draw inspiration from the wisdom found in Scripture. Proverbs 4:23 reminds us to guard our hearts, for everything we do flows from it.

In your *Heart Journey*™ *Journal* Heartwork for this segment, you will explore and define the values that you aspire to embody in your relationships.

## FOUR HORSEMEN AND THEIR ANTIDOTES

Renowned for their expertise in marriage and family counseling, Drs. John and Julie Gottman present the concept of the four horsemen of the apocalypse in relationships. These horsemen, namely criticism, defensiveness, contempt, and stonewalling, can wreak havoc on our connections with others. Now, with much of our heart home healthy, walking in right relationships and staying out of criticism, defensiveness, contempt, and stonewalling, will be our objective. We will use the antidotes to the horsemen as well as Scriptures that can help us counteract their negative influence.[36]

Instead of resorting to criticism, which involves being judgmental and fault-finding, we should strive for a gentle startup in our conversations. Using the phrase "the story I make up is…" can provide a non-threatening way to address concerns. By giving each other grace as we work through the situation, we can decrease both the tendency to criticize others and our own defensiveness. Proverbs 15:1 (NIV) reminds us that "a gentle answer turns away wrath."

When faced with defensiveness, it is essential to take responsibility for our own part in the conflict. Rather than reacting defensively, we should aim to describe our own feelings and needs. This approach promotes understanding and empathy, fostering healthier communication. Psalm 51:10 encourages us to pray for a clean heart and a renewed spirit, enabling us to respond with humility and self-reflection.

Contempt, a toxic emotion that arises from a sense of superiority, must be countered with respect and kindness. Contempt is a relationship assassin. By focusing on expressing our own emotions and needs, we can avoid belittling or demeaning our loved ones. Colossians 3:12 reminds us to clothe ourselves with compassion, kindness, humility, gentleness, and patience, fostering an environment of love and respect.

Stonewalling, a defensive mechanism characterized by shutting down and withdrawing, can be overcome through self-soothing techniques. Rather than suppressing emotions, we can learn to manage our internal turmoil in healthy ways. Seeking solace in prayer and finding inner peace can help us maintain open and constructive communication. Avoidance kills relationships, causing a slow drifting away from one another. In Matthew 5:23-24, Jesus teaches that before presenting our gifts to God, we should first communicate honestly with each other, clearing up conflict rather than ignoring it. This implies that stonewalling is contrary to God's principle of resolving issues and fostering honest relationships.

## POSITIVE SENTIMENT OVERRIDE

In their research, the Gottmans also emphasize the importance of positive sentiment override in relationships. This involves interpreting and responding to situations in a positive light, fostering a positive sense of joy and connection. By creating enjoyable experiences and focusing on shared activities, we can cultivate a positive atmosphere that outweighs the negative. In addition, we want to strive to express appreciation and affirmation regularly, creating an environment of positivity and love. Proverbs 16:24 reminds us that gracious words are like honey, sweet to the soul and healing to the bones. We must focus on the positive in each other.

Open your *Heart Journey™ Journal* to Chapter Eleven and complete your **Individual Heartwork - Navigating Relationship Anew,** and enjoy this activity: **God-Filled Relationships Activity.**

Use this QR code to access audible versions of activities.

Beloved, wow, you astonish me—look at all you have accomplished!

We have one more chapter to go. In Chapter Twelve, we will wrap up our journey with some consolidative healing activities, and we will celebrate all God has done. Oh, dear one, what an honor it is to stride with you, both in the valleys and on the mountain tops!

## LET US PRAY.

*Heavenly Father,*

*I pray that You would help us to incorporate everything we have learned on this journey and to move forward in purpose. Thank You for all the healing and for giving us the grace to become all You have made us to be.*

*In Jesus' name, Amen.*

# *Chapter*
## TWELVE
### Restoring My Life

*Wait and listen, everyone who is thirsty! Come to the waters; and he who has no money, come, buy and eat! Yes, come, buy [priceless, spiritual] wine and milk without money and without price [simply for the self-surrender that accepts the blessing].*

*Why do you spend your money for that which is not bread, and your earnings for what does not satisfy? Hearken diligently to Me, and eat what is good, and let your soul delight itself in fatness [the profuseness of spiritual joy].*

*Incline your ear [submit and consent to the divine will] and come to Me; hear, and your soul will revive; and I will make an everlasting covenant or league with you, even the sure mercy (kindness, goodwill, and compassion) promised to David.*

Isaiah 55:1-3 (AMPC)

Beloved, here we stand together, our hearts holding hands, at the culmination of your profound journey toward healing. As we bring this transformative study to a close, I am overcome with emotion, for we have trod upon sacred ground, embarking on a path less traveled together. Just as my late father longed for the solace of his ashes to be laid in the heart of Waipi'o Valley, beneath the majestic Hi'ilawe Falls, we, too, have ventured into uncharted territory.

As our hearts have returned home to belonging, permit me, if you would, to take you on one of my journeys to one of my home states, Hawai'i, to the Big Island.

## THE SACRED KING'S PATH

Hi'ilawe Falls, renowned for its towering height of 1,450 feet and its enchanting cascade, stands as the crown jewel of Waipi'o Valley on the north end of the Big Island of Hawai'i. This valley, aptly named the "Valley of the Kings," is carved deeply into the embrace of Kohala Mountain, boasting awe-inspiring cliffs that reach 3,000 feet into the heavens. The valley's grandeur is further enhanced by the presence of the sublime and ever-moving Waipi'o River. Throughout centuries, Hawaiian ali'i, the noble rulers, called this valley their permanent home, and the remnants of the King's Path can still be discovered amidst its sacred cliffs and valleys.

To journey in to Hi'ilawe Falls is to embark on a treacherous path, one that demands special permissions, bodily rigor, and unparalleled courage. Yet, the elation that floods your being upon reaching its hidden depths and emerging back to the shores of the powerful deep blue ocean breaking against the black sand shore is nothing short of extraordinary and other-worldly. Undoubtedly, such an endeavor comes at a significant cost—a price paid in courage, determination, and audacity. It demands the investment of an entire day, traversing through moments of uncertainty and the physical toll of sweat, perhaps even tears, and the inevitable cuts and bruises along the way. Yet, despite the challenges, my earthly father deemed this price worthwhile, recognizing that the reward far surpassed the sacrifices made.

And so, your *Heart Journey*™ mirrors this sacred pilgrimage. The reverence that resonates within Waipi'o Valley, cherished by the Hawaiian people as a hallowed place, intertwines with the essence of our own quest. We have traversed sacred ground, scaling mountains and venturing into valleys, following the meandering path of the river, at times gentle and tranquil, at others fierce and relentless. Yet, we have discovered the King's Path, leading us back to the "Valley of the Kings," where every facet of our being finds solace and fulfillment, akin to Mephibosheth feasting at the King's table.

Our journey, guided by a profound sense of purpose, has not been without its challenges. We encountered obstacles along the winding river, and uncertainty occasionally clouded our path. However, with each step and struggle, we pressed onward, fortified by an unwavering devotion to our Heavenly Father.

Our expedition, akin to the breathtaking Waipi'o Valley, beautifully encapsulates both the exhilaration and challenges that accompany the quest for its double hidden waterfall within the royal home of the King. The Hi'ilawe Falls, with its cascading double waterfalls, mirrors the abundant flow of our King's double flow of living water that now issues forth from the very places we have suffered deep wounding. Under the double flow of living water, we have discovered that the King has a divine plan for each one of us that surpasses our wildest dreams. Moreover, our fierce journey has granted us special access to the inner chambers of the King's heart, and we have abided with Him. Like Adam and Eve, we walked with him in the garden of the King's Valley under the double flow of grace. It was here that we have laid down our ashes of trauma, wounding, anxiety, and resentment and received in exchange, profuse beauty and purpose in this awe-inspiring dwelling of the King (Isaiah 61:3). In seeking to enter His royal home,

He has also infiltrated the dark places of our heart home, restoring all that has been lost.

As I sit here writing this chapter to you, tears streaming down my face, I am acutely aware of the extraordinary achievement you have realized. You have accomplished something that only few dare to undertake. Many around us may choose to take a spiritual bypass, avoiding the inner renovation work required to heal, grow, and become, using salvation as an excuse to linger at the shore and never venture into the double portion in the King's Valley. But you have embraced the arduous and sacrificial path of transformation with unwavering commitment to His purpose. Your love for Him is evident, Beloved. And you have responded to the Lord's call in Isiah 66:1 (NIV), "Where is the house you will build for Me? Where will My resting place be?" You have allowed every nook and cranny of your heart home to become His delightful repose.

In the depth of your being, you have confronted the shadows, faced your fears, illuminated the quivering recesses of your heart, and allowed the most vulnerable parts of your heart home to be seen and loved. Your willingness to journey with Him into the core of your being is a testament to your courage, strength, and unyielding faith. You have chosen to navigate the complexities of your inner landscape, unearthing the very treasure of Jesus, who now beams more brightly from your mended being. Together, our heart homes have become a group of renovated dazzling abodes that form a bright city on the King's mountain (Matthew 5:14).

For those of you who have journeyed alongside a friend or with a small group, I celebrate the profound connections forged in the crucible of vulnerability and shared healing. These relationships have grown stronger, fortified by the unbreakable bond we form when we face our deepest wounds together. You have called each other deeper into the King's Valley as you tenderly nursed each other's punctures and bruises along the way to double portion. This indeed is the holy ground of love that Jesus yearned for when He beseeched, "I pray for them all to be joined together as one even as You and I, Father, are joined together as one. I pray for them to become one with us" (John 17:21, TPT). This kind of vulnerability requires courage and yields an abundant recompense.

## THE ARENA

Theodore Roosevelt once spoke of the courageous souls who dare to step into the arena of the fight. He emphasized that it is not the critic, but the one who strives valiantly, with a face marred by dust, sweat, and blood, who deserves credit. This individual embraces both triumph and failure, for there is no worthy effort without errors or shortcomings. They are driven by great enthusiasms and unwavering devotions, dedicating themselves to a noble cause. Even in the face of potential defeat, they dare greatly, ensuring that their place shall never be among the cold and timid souls who never tasted victory or experienced defeat. You have stepped courageously into the arena of the King's Valley, imperfectly fighting your way through, to emerge victorious with a double portion. You have embraced the challenges, faced your fears, and triumphed over the adversary.

## THE SEED OF SALVATION WITHIN TRAUMA

Beloved, in this sacred and victorious moment, I ask that together we transverse into the "Valley of the King" one more time, and peer into Jesus' final days on Earth through the lens of trauma. Let us zoom in on Jesus' greatest earthly act—the act that reversed the curse and irrevocably altered the course of history ... the betrayal, scourging, and crucifixion of Jesus.

Our freedom came at an unfathomable cost—a trauma that reverberated not only through Jesus Himself, but also through the very souls of His mother and closest friends. Picture, if you will, the searing pain etched upon the face of His mother as she witnessed her beloved Son being ruthlessly and mercilessly murdered. While we now understand that Jesus willingly laid down His life, we cannot overlook the profound trauma that gripped Mary's mother's heart. In the depths of her being, it was an anguish that tore through her soul, leaving behind scars that would forever bear witness to her profound loss.

And then there was Peter, dear Peter, who, in the midst of the Lord's trauma, denied any association with Him. Oh, the weight of that moment! It deepened the wounds within Peter's heart, inflicting what we refer to as moral injury—an injury born out of the betrayal of one's own moral compass. Can you imagine the tumultuous storm that raged within Peter's spirit? The inner turmoil, the haunting whispers of guilt and regret that pierced his conscience? His denial became a stark reminder of the frailty and vulnerability of human nature in the face of overwhelming trauma.

Moreover, the disciples, as a collective, endured a different kind of anguish—a community trauma that shattered the very foundations of their existence. Their leader, their guide, was ripped away from them in the most brutal and heinous manner imaginable. Can you feel the tendrils of terror and confusion entwining their hearts? The anguish of witnessing their beloved friend and mentor being ripped from their midst, leaving them grappling with a colossal betrayal and the tragic loss of a dear companion? And to compound their pain, in the midst of their community trauma, one of their own succumbed to the overwhelming weight of despair and chose to end their own life. Oh, the depths of their grief, the fractures that splintered his sense of belonging and security!

And yet, my Beloved, within this extraordinary trauma lay the seed of salvation for the world. Can you fathom the remarkable beauty that emerged from the depths of suffering? As we contemplate our affinity for stories like "Beauty and the Beast," let us delve deeper into their resonance within our souls. We are drawn to these tales because they embody our longing for the reversal of curses within our own lives and lands. And truly, through this ultimate trauma, the curse was overturned, and salvation was bestowed upon the world (Galatians 3:13).

The adversary, in His relentless pursuit, sought to beat, brutalize, and extinguish the very essence of the Son of God. Yet little did he know that God, in his boundless wisdom, had meticulously crafted a plan—a plan that would transform the vilest of evils into the wellspring of redemption and salvation. At the deepest crevasse of the horrific trauma, the King's corpse bowed silent on the cross. The spear was gouged into His side, and the double flow of blood and water forcefully gushed out, lavishing beauty for ashes upon the world.

Oh, my Beloved, find solace in the knowledge that God is weaving a similar masterpiece within your own life. He takes every ounce of pain, every deep-seated wound, and every searing trauma, and carefully weaves them together into goodness that surpasses measure.

Beloved, God is working in your life, transforming it into a place of beauty, reversing the curse. You are rising in every place of wound through the brightness of resurrection power in the King. And through His divine interventions, He will continue to heal you. As we conclude this study, let us underline the significance of seeking continual encounters with Jesus and being filled with the Holy Spirit. Jesus said in John 14:21 (ESV), "Whoever has My commandments and keeps them, he it is who loves Me. And he who loves Me will be loved by My Father, and I will love him and manifest Myself to him." He will manifest Himself to you as you seek Him, Beloved.

## LAVISH RESTORATION

The Scripture declares in Acts 2:17 (NIV), "In the last days, God says, 'I will pour out My Spirit on all people. Your sons and daughters will prophesy, your young men will see visions, your old men will dream dreams.'"

With this in mind, permit me to share a dream that I believe was bestowed upon me. This dream was distinct from my ordinary dream life, as if it were a heavenly gift. In the dream, I found myself carefree as a child, running through a room with endlessly high ceilings. Layers upon layers of soft, white, beautiful fabric hung from the ceiling, allowing me to run for miles, my hand gliding across the fabric, just as a child would playfully run through a clothesline. Upon awakening, I sought the Lord for the dream's interpretation. Upon searching the Scriptures, I discovered that white signifies purification, the deeds of the Saints, and various forms of restoration and sanctification. I believe the meaning behind this dream is that boundless purity and restoration are available to us, and we can receive them with childlike openness.

Around the same period, my husband and I purchased a home that was to be built. We were unaware of the name of the road we would call home at that time, but later discovered that our house would be situated on Restoration Drive. Once again, my thoughts turned to the dream, and I felt the Lord was speaking to me that He offers extravagantly abundant restoration and purpose to His people.

And what is He saying to you amidst all this? I believe He is inviting you to abide within the Valley of Kings, to a heart home marked by restoration, where more and more lavish renewal and refreshing awaits you. You can join Him on the royal King's Path at any moment, feast at His table, and embrace an abundance of white linen—purification, restoration, and purposeful deeds—uniquely designed for you, lavishly bestowed upon you. Here, you are home. And He is saying, "Come and drink," as Isaiah 55 proclaims, for there is more than enough, flowing from His double waterfall of restoration. You now abide more deeply in Him, and He abides in you, in every room of your renewed heart home. Welcome home to belonging, Beloved. The abode of the King is within you.

Furthermore, this is just the beginning of many more opportunities for healing your heart home. I am thrilled to announce that Restoration Media, LLC also publishes a series of *Heart Journey*™ studies, offering profound exploration and impartation of each aspect of the healing process: Stability, Rewrite, Restore, Relate, and Launch, all written from my heart to yours. These studies provide a deeper understanding and guidance for your own personal journey toward healing in and through him.

As we reach the conclusion of this study, I want you to know that I believe in you and in Him within you. Let your pursuit of restoration be a constant journey, intimately entwined with Him as you walk hand in hand with Him along the King's Path, which is established within you. Embrace the truth of your royal identity, knowing that you are profoundly loved and cherished by Him, and walk confidently in your divine purpose as His adored queen, whose home is His belonging. And Beloved, I will be with you soon you in the next *Heart Journey*™ study, and in the meanwhile, I, too, will be walking with Him in the Valley of the King.

Open your *Heart Journey Journal* one last time for your **Individual Heartwork - Restoring My Life.**

And enjoy the scripted activities from our study at any time by submitting your best email here:

## LET US PRAY.

*Heavenly Father,*

*May we embrace the restoration that arises from the depths of suffering, just as salvation emerged from the ultimate trauma. May we lay down all ashes for the King's double portion of splendor. May we trust in God's meticulous plan, knowing that He weaves together every pain and wound into a tapestry of immeasurable good. And may we seek continual encounters with Jesus, being filled with the Holy Spirit, as we embark on Your journey of restoration and purpose.*

*In Jesus' name, Amen.*

# References

[1] Christian persecution higher than ever as Open Doors' World Watch List marks 30 years." Religion News. January 17, 2023. Retrieved from https://religionnews.com/2023/01/17/christian-persecution-higher-than-ever-as-open-doors-world-watch-list-marks-30-years/

[2] Miller, W. R., & Delaney, H. D. (Eds.). (2005). Judeo-Christian perspectives on psychology: Human nature, motivation, and change. American Psychological Association.hIps://doi.org/10.1037/10859-000

[3] Netburn, D. (2023, January 9). Group therapy from the pulpit? How a professor and minister is changing psychology. Los Angeles Times. Retrieved from hIps://www.la'mes.com/california/story/2023-01-09/psychologistand-minister-thema-bryant.

[4] See "Disclaimer" on page 19.

[5] "Heart" in Logos Factbook, (Logos Bible Software, 2021), accessed March 9, 2023, https://app.logos.com/factbook/christianity.jesus-christ.

[6] Deborah is an Alias. Please note that all the stories and characters depicted in this book are entirely fictional and do not represent any actual person, living or deceased, with the exception of Deborah (alias), who has consented to the author sharing her experiences following the *Heart Journey*™ Method. This book does not feature any representation of clients from the author's psychotherapy practice.

[7] Baumrind, D. (2013). Authoritative parenting revisited: History and current status. In R. E. Larzelere, A. Sheffield, & A. W. Harrist (Eds.), Authoritative parenting: Synthesizing nurturance and discipline for optimal child development.

[8] Smith, S. D. (2017). Sacred rest: Recover your life, renew your energy, restore your sanity. FaithWords.

[9] "Interoception" is a term coined by Dan Siegel, MD.

[10] Grounding and Tracking skills come from the somatic psychotherapies. whose father is generally said to be Peter Levine.

[11] "We should fix ourselves firmly in the presence of God by conversing all the time with Him...in this conversation of the soul with God, we are not even required to speak much or to think much, provided we acknowledge ourselves as inferior to Him and as dependent upon Him in everything."- Brother Lawrence. "The Practice of the Presence of God." Translated by John Delaney. Doubleday, 1977.

[12] It is important to note that recognizing the nurturing qualities of Jesus does not mean turning God into a female. God is beyond gender and encompasses all characteristics of both male and female (Genesis 1:27). The use of maternal language is simply a way to better understand the depth and intimacy of God's love for us. As we embrace this aspect of God's nature, we can internalize a greater sense of wholeness and healing through our relationship with Him.

[13] Linnemann, A., Kappert, M. B., Fischer, S., Doerr, J. M., Strahler, J., & Nater, U. M. (2015). The effects of music listening on pain and stress in the daily life of patients with fibromyalgia syndrome. Frontiers in Human Neuroscience, 9, 434. https://doi.org/10.3389/fnhum.2015.00434

[14] While the concept of Dialectic of Acceptance and Seeking Change is found in the scriptures, Marsha Linehan also defines and uses this concept in her Dialectical Behavioral Therapy Method. Linehan, M. M. (2014). DBT® Skills Training Handouts and Worksheets, Second Edition. The Guilford Press.

[15] Titration is from the somatic trauma healing arenas and originates with Peter Levine. Levine, P. A. (1997). Waking the Tiger: Healing Trauma. North Atlantic Books.

[16] Working the edges is from the somatic healing trauma areanas and originates with Peter Levine. Levine, P. A. (1997). Waking the Tiger: Healing Trauma. North Atlantic Books.

[17] Ecker, B., (2020). Erasing Problematic Emotional Learnings: Psychotherapeutic Use of Memory Reconsolidation Research. In Lane, R. D., & Nadel, L. (Eds), Neuroscience of Enduring Change Implications for Psychotherapy (pp. 273-299). Oxford. https://doi.org/10.1176/appi.psychotherapy.20200052

[18] "Over-and-Under-Coupling" is from the somatic healing trauma arena and originates with Peter Levine. Levine, P. A. (1997). Waking the Tiger: Healing Trauma. North Atlantic Books.

[19] Pennebaker, J. W., & Seagal, J. D. (1999). Forming a story: The health benefits of narrative. Journal of Clinical Psychology, 55(10), 1243–1254. https://doi.org/10.1002/(SICI)1097-4679(199910)55:10<1243::AID-JCLP6>3.0.CO;2-N

[20] Van der Kolk, B. A. (2015). The body keeps the score: Brain, mind, and body in the healing of trauma. Penguin Books.

[21] Ecker, B., (2020). Erasing Problematic Emotional Learnings: Psychotherapeutic Use of Memory Reconsolidation Research. In Lane, R. D., & Nadel, L. (Eds), Neuroscience of Enduring Change: Implications for Psychotherapy (pp.273-299). Oxford. https://doi.org/10.1176/appi.psychotherapy.20200052z

[22] Schwartz, R. C. (2013). Internal Family Systems therapy (2nd ed.). The Guilford Press; Young, J. E., Klosko, J. S., & Weishaar, M. E. (2003). Schema therapy: A practitioner's guide. Guilford Press.

[23] Brown, B. (2007). I thought it was just me (but it isn't): Telling the truth about perfectionism, inadequacy, and power. Penguin.

[24] Wells, G. L., & Olson, E. A. (2003). Eyewitness testimony. Annual Review of Psychology, 54, 277-295. https://doi.org/10.1146/annurev.psych.54.101601.145028

[25] Berntsen, D., & Rubin, D. C. (2006). The centrality of event scale: A measure of integrating a trauma into one's identity and its relation to post-traumatic stress disorder symptoms. Behaviour Research and Therapy, 44(2), 219-231. https://doi.org/10.1016/j.brat.2005.01.009

[26] Lehrner, A. & Yehuda, R. (2018). Cultural trauma and epigenetic inheritance. Development and Psychopathology, 30(5), 1763-1777. doi: 10.1017/S0954579418001153.

[27] Levine, P. A. (2010). In an unspoken voice: How the body releases trauma and restores goodness. North Atlantic Books.

[28] Witvliet, C. V., Ludwig, T. E., & Vander Laan, K. L. (2001). Granting forgiveness or harboring grudges: Implications for emotion, physiology, and health. Psychological Science, 12(2), 117–123. https://doi.org/10.1111/1467-9280.00320

[29] Toussaint, L. L., & Webb, J. R. (2005). Gender differences in the relationship between empathy and forgiveness. Journal of Social Psychology, 145(6), 673–685. https://doi.org/10.3200/SOCP.145.6.673-685

[30] Worthington, E. L., Witvliet, C. V., Pietrini, P., & Miller, A. J. (2011). Forgiveness, health, and well-being: A review of evidence for emotional versus decisional forgiveness, dispositional forgivingness, and reduced unforgiveness. Journal of behavioral medicine, 34(4), 270-280.

[31] Foster, R. J. (2018). Celebration of Discipline, Special Anniversary Edition: The Path to Spiritual Growth – Special Edition. Harper One.

[32] Price, C. (2021). The Power of Fun: How to Feel Alive Again. The Dial Press.

[33] Hebb, D. O. (1949). The organization of behavior: A neuropsychological theory. Wiley.

[34] Fredrickson, B. L. (2013). Love 2.0: Creating Happiness and Health in Moments of Connection. Plume.

[35] Real, T. (2008, January 29). The New Rules of Marriage: What You Need to Know to Make Love Work. Ballantine Books.

[36] Gottman, J., & Silver, N. (2015). The Seven Principles for Making Marriage Work: A Practical Guide from the Country's Foremost Relationship Expert. Harmony.

Made in the USA
Columbia, SC
14 August 2023